FIRST-TIME PREGNANCY GUIDE *For Moms*

What to Expect During Pregnancy and Childbirth

Gina Wing RN, BSN, PHN

GINA WING RN, BSN, PHN

Printed in the United States of America
First Printing 2022
First Edition 2022

1 0 9 8 7 6 5 4 3 2 1

Disclaimer

The content in this guidebook is meant for information purposes only. It is important that our readers do their own research and work with healthcare professionals before making any decisions about their health, to ensure their pregnancy and delivery are taken care of according to their needs. The reader should take independent healthcare advice from a professional in connection with, or independently research and verify, any information that they find in this guidebook before relying on it, whether it is for a decision related to pregnancy and delivery or not. The goal of this book is to provide the reader with the resources they need to plan their pregnancy and be prepared for giving birth. Always get professional help to put your plan in motion.

Dedication

To the many nurses, physicians and CNM's I've had the pleasure to work with over the last 25 years. I am humbled to be working amongst some of the best!

And to my patients that I've had the pleasure of caring for ~ YOU are the reason for my passion in Labor & Delivery. Thank you for allowing me to be a part of your birth story.

Table of Contents

Introduction

Having a baby is exciting and rewarding, but a lot of work. It's a wonderful experience, but parenthood can also be tiring. The best thing to do is prepare as much as possible.

If you are reading this book prior to getting pregnant, you are merely giving yourself a head start on thinking ahead, and careful planning only sets you up for success. If you find yourself already pregnant and anticipating what's to come congratulations! I commend you as well for taking the steps to understand what lies ahead for you and your baby.

Back in 1991, I found myself pregnant and overjoyed. By the end of my pregnancy, I had relocated to the central coast of California and found myself now going to be a single mom. I was a young 23-year-old but determined to continue living my best life, and give my son the best life I could. Naturally, as most newly pregnant moms do, I did my share of research and educated myself on what was to come. I remember it as being very black-and-white. You must do this. You must not do that.

I eventually had my son, and two years later enrolled in college to become a nurse. A labor nurse to be exact. Yes, my labor nurse "Sparky" had that much of an impact on me. She was the absolute best! She was my nurse three days in a row and I was determined to make that kind of impact on other moms' lives for years to come.

I actually loved being pregnant so much that I agreed to be a surrogate mom for a friend that was unable to bear children of her own. I must say this was one of the most rewarding things I've ever done in my life.

I eventually went on to remarry and found myself in the throes of infertility. After struggling to get pregnant we embarked on the IVF journey since I knew it worked two times prior with my surrogacy pregnancies. After getting pregnant, we suffered a miscarriage at 14 weeks. It was devastating, to say the least.

As a labor nurse for 25 years now, I've shared in the many, many joys of childbirth with women of all ages, races, ethnicities, and values. The unfortunate side of being a labor nurse is also having to share in the heartbreak of losses.

My hope as you read along is that you can understand a bit better what is to come, what everything that is happening to you and your body means, as well as help you embrace the amazingness of what our bodies are made to do. Some things you might not want to hear, you might disagree with or you might just think I'm being a little harsh in how I explain things.

It is my personality to be very blunt and to the point. Please realize my intention in writing this is only to help further educate you by explaining things in a clear, concise manner; the way I wish they were explained to me prior to becoming a nurse.

1

Choosing Your Healthcare Provider

Medical science has thankfully progressed by leaps and bounds over the past two centuries, and the possible risks around pregnancy and childbirth have been greatly minimized. That is, under the care and attention of qualified medical professionals. There's a reason why obstetrics (a branch of medicine and surgery that focuses on childbirth), gynecology (a branch of medicine concerned with female health, including pregnancy), and midwifery are specializations and not something just anyone takes care of. Choosing who gets the honor of assisting you on this amazing journey may seem daunting, but I'll help you determine what you should look for in a great OB-GYN (obstetrician-gynecologist), midwife, and others who may be involved with your new blossoming family.

Enjoying Your Pregnancy

A healthy mom usually means a healthy pregnancy. There are some exceptions of course, but meeting with your care provider prior to getting pregnant is optimal for identifying any risks you might have and discussing any health concerns you might have. Having your partner attend this first appointment can be helpful as well, as they also have a family medical history and possible risks that can also affect your baby.

Choosing an OB-GYN and/or Midwife

It's important to know that you don't have to settle for the first option that crosses your path. The right OB-GYN or midwife for your best friend/cousin/sister might not be the right one for you. That doesn't mean they're a bad OB-GYN or midwife, there are simply more factors to consider other than just skill if you want to make the most of this experience.

Difference between an OB-GYN and a midwife

Both OB-GYNs and midwives are qualified health professionals that provide prenatal (before birth and related to pregnancy), pregnancy, birth, and postpartum (after birth) care. Each path has its own specialized training and certification, and different areas of expertise. Although they both work in the same field, their education is different. OB-GYNs are medical doctors who specialize in female reproductive health, pregnancy, and delivery.

In the US, there are three levels of midwife credentials. Some midwives are licensed while others are not. Some work in birth centers or hospitals while others only work within your home. The CNM or Certified Nurse Midwife is a nurse midwife who is certified by the International Federation of Midwives. A CNM is an advanced practice registered nurse who has completed registered nursing and midwifery education. They are credentialed as a Certified Nurse Midwife and regulated by the Board of Registered Nursing.

There's also a CM Certified Midwife which is a midwife who is certified by the American Midwifery Certification Board (AMCB). The certified midwife does not require a nursing degree but does include the same information in midwifery and women's health as the CNM program.

You also have a Traditional Birth Attendant (TBA) which is also known as Traditional Midwives, Community Midwives, or Lay Midwives. These midwives are not credentialed and may not have received formal training or education. TBAs are not regulated and there's no registration.

Does your health insurance cover them?

Unfortunately, this is a reality that we have to face, not all OB-GYNs and midwives may be covered by your health insurance. So, before you commit to someone and become attached, check that your insurance will cover the bill. There's no need to add financial stress to the list of things to consider. This is as simple as going to your insurance provider's website and checking the list of OB-GYNs and midwives that they cover.

Ask around

Friends and Family

Never underestimate the power of word-of-mouth. You can of course ask close friends and family members for recommendations! Personal testimony is often the most useful indicator of the type of care you'll receive, instead of a list of qualifications and awards. Your closest friends and family are also likely to know you very well and are most likely to guide you in the direction of the right OB-GYN or midwife for you. Others who have already experienced pregnancy and childbirth will also know what to look out for in terms of things they wished they'd known, things they would've done differently, and care providers they wished they'd gone to see instead. Hindsight is 20/20 after all. As I stated before, one provider might be perfect for one person, and far from it for the other. Your best bet is to pick a few choices that have good reputations and go for the first visit with each. Have a list of questions that are important to you and write down your answers so you remember them. Do they align with your beliefs and your desires? How many days and weekends are they on call? Do they deliver or use OB hospitalists which means you probably won't see them at all for delivery? You also want to be sure and look up everyone's C-section record. Just because you might come in contact with an all-woman practice does not mean that they all do what is right for all women. Sad, but true.

Forums

We now live in a time and place where you can also ask strangers on the internet for advice. There are hundreds of forums for prospective moms where you can chat about your personal journey, your experiences, ask and answer questions, and just generally get support. Some questions are just easier to ask anonymously from strangers, aren't they? Particularly the awkward ones. Some of the best forums at the time of writing are:

- Momtastic Pregnancy Forum: https://pregnancyforum.momtastic.com/
- Keep Em Cookin Forum: http://forum.keepemcookin.com/
- Reddit r/pregnant: https://www.reddit.com/r/pregnant/
- Parenting Forums Pregnancy: https://www.parentingforums.org/forums/pregnancy.3/

And best of all, if you have unique health concerns, there are forums created specifically for you! Such as:

- Diabetes Forum Pregnancy: https://www.diabetes.co.uk/forum/category/pregnancy.47/

- Health Unlocked Pregnancy and mental health concerns: https://community.whattoexpect.com/forums/mental-health-disorders-and-pregnancy.html

All you need to do is search and you will find a community that can provide you with advice suited to your needs.

Please don't forget that you pick your OB provider for a reason, because they align with your desires and wishes, and you trust them. The last thing you want to do is get a bunch of information from the internet and presume anything. There's a lot of great info out there but there's also a lot of bad info. Instead of assuming everything you read on the internet is accurate, make a list of questions that you have with things you've read and clarify information at your appointments. Either what you're reading is correct, or is a little off, or can be completely wrong. Your practitioner should be able to explain things further and put your mind at ease.

Reviews

An added benefit of the internet is that every healthcare provider can now be reviewed by their clients. A quick Google search of the specific OB-GYN or midwife you have in mind will provide you with a star rating out of five, as well as any Google reviews clients have left. This is another good way of getting feedback on others' experiences and whether they had any concerns. An OB-GYN or midwife with a poor rating is best to be avoided. Of course, if there's only one bad review then possibly a client just had a bad experience. Take it with a grain of salt if all the other reviews are great.

You can also check the overall rating of the hospital you are considering for your delivery as patients leave reviews of their overall experience of the care they received, regardless of the reason for their stay, the friendliness of the staff who work there, how quickly concerns were addressed and help was received. If you are dead set on a hospital, you might look to make sure the practitioner you have chosen practices at that hospital. Not all physicians and midwives practice at every hospital even if it's in the same vicinity.

Check their qualifications and location

This might seem self-explanatory, but it's always good to check an OB-GYN's and midwife's board certification and what specialties, history, and experience they have under their belt. You might want an OB-GYN who specializes in patients with high blood pressure because you have a family history or a midwife who specializes in water births.

And of course, it doesn't help if your dream OB-GYN or midwife practices on the other side of the country, even if you are willing to fly for every consultation. It's important to have someone relatively close in case of emergencies. If you live in a rural area, you might have fewer options available close to you, but at least make plans for who can be accessed in the shortest amount of time. Some soon-to-be-parents prefer a specific hospital for the delivery and then will choose an OB-GYN or midwife that delivers at that particular facility.

Are they the care provider for you?

Something first-time parents might not always think about is whether the OB-GYN or midwife of your choice suits you personally. This includes their consultation style, are they warm and gentle, or are they more clinical and serious? Are they male or female? Because yes, this does play a role in your preferences. There is no evidence that male OB-GYNs perform poorer than female OB-GYNs, but approximately 60% of female patients prefer a female OB-GYN. If that doesn't matter to you, feel free to pick an OB-GYN of any gender. Nearly 99% of midwives in the USA are however female, so finding a male midwife will be tricky, should that be your preference.

Where do you want to give birth?

Do you want to give birth in a hospital or have a home delivery? C-section or natural birth? There are pros and cons to all of these, which will be discussed in more detail in chapter 4, *Delivery Time*. It's important to be open and upfront with all your wishes with your chosen healthcare professional, as this will enable them to provide you with the best advice and care suited to your needs. Both OB-GYNs and midwives work in hospitals, but only OB-GYNs can perform C-sections. CMs can assist with home births, and also practice in freestanding birth centers unaffiliated with a hospital. Although some hospitals do accommodate water labors/births under the care of an OB-GYN, they are still most commonly under the care of midwives. High-risk pregnancies are strongly recommended to be managed by OB-GYNs in a hospital setting, as this is the safest and most controlled environment where any eventualities can be handled correctly (more on pregnancies in chapter 3, *What To Expect, The Good, The Bad, and Staying Healthy*).

Should your healthcare provider advise against something in your plans regarding your pregnancy and delivery, for example recommending a hospital birth over a home birth, don't disregard them immediately. Consider *why* they are giving this advice. For example, if you've dreamed of a home delivery, but find out you're expecting twins, it's in your best interest to listen if your OB-GYN or midwife suggests a hospital delivery instead. If you truly don't agree with them, you're always welcome to choose a different healthcare provider, but most often they're simply trying to give you the best options for the best outcomes for you and your baby.

Doulas

Sometimes there's nothing greater than having a doula there to be your guide and support during labor. A doula is someone who fills the role of a supporting companion during childbirth, by making their client feel safe and comfortable, and by giving advice.

How is a doula different from a midwife?

Doulas are trained professionals, however, they're not healthcare professionals and don't have any healthcare qualifications like nurses, midwives, or OB-GYNs. Generally, doulas don't perform deliveries but provide emotional support, care, and information to the expecting parent. Pregnancy and birth are already physically and emotionally taxing, especially if it's your first time, so having someone kind and knowledgeable around can make a huge difference.

Picking a doula

Should you consider the services of a doula, make sure to interview them, get references from other clients they've assisted, check their reputation, and above all, make sure that they are the doula that suits your personal needs. It's important that both of you understand that they are not your primary healthcare provider when it comes to your pregnancy and delivery. OB-GYNs, midwives, and nurses have years of education and experience that can help you and your baby stay safe while in the hospital, whereas a doula is there to provide support.

A doula should not make decisions for you or pressure you to go against the advice of your healthcare providers. Doulas don't have any formal education in obstetrics, which can in some cases mean they might not be as educated regarding treatments and medication.

Some cases I've experienced as a labor and delivery nurse include a doula who convinced a patient not to take antibiotics, even though she had GBS (Group Beta Strep) infection. If passed to the infant, GBS can have devastating and even fatal consequences.

Another example is a doula who tried to prevent the use of Pitocin in a patient's IV after delivery, even though the patient was actively bleeding. It is totally understandable if a patient would like to not have Pitocin after delivery if they are not bleeding. However, if you are actively bleeding there are only a few things that will help it stop. Personally, I'd rather have a little Pitocin in my IV to stop my bleeding rather than need a blood transfusion due to too much blood loss.

Don't let these examples scare you off though, not all doulas are pushy with their own agenda. It's always important to be as informed and as prepared as possible. We should be all on the same team, working toward the goal of a healthy mama and a healthy baby.

Family medicine doctors

Some family medicine doctors can provide you with care during your pregnancy, delivery, and postpartum care.

However, it's important to consult them first on whether they provide pregnancy care, and whether they're qualified to perform C-sections, as not all family medicine doctors have undergone the training. If you have a family medicine doctor who ticks all the boxes and you would prefer that they be the primary healthcare professional on your journey, make an appointment with them to discuss your options.

Trust your instincts

At the end of the day, it's all down to you to make an informed, educated decision that suits you. You are the one who will be carrying a baby and giving birth. If something about your healthcare provider rubs you and/or your partner the wrong way, trust your instincts and switch to someone more suitable. You don't have to stick with someone just because you've seen them for one or two appointments, or because they came highly recommended. This is *your* experience and you can take charge of it.

Summary

To summarize everything that's been discussed in this chapter to help you make an informed decision, I've compiled all the information in this table for comparison.

	OB-GYN	Midwife	Doula	Family medicine doctor
Is a medical professional	+	+	-	+
Can perform C-sections	+	-	-	Only if specifically trained
Can manage high-risk pregnancies	+	-	-	Only if specifically trained
Can manage low-risk pregnancies	+	+	-	Confirm with your family medicine doctor
Can deliver in a hospital	+	+	-	-
Can provide home delivery	-	+	-	+
Can provide water birth	In select hospitals	+	-	Confirm with your family medicine doctor
Can prescribe medication	+	Only if they are a CNM	-	+
Provides prenatal, birth, and postpartum support	+	+	+	Confirm with your family medicine doctor

2

Becoming Pregnant

Now that you've made the decision that you want to start a family, you probably want to work on getting pregnant. But what if you're on birth control? What if you have a health condition like diabetes? What if you have a family history of infertility? If you're already pregnant, you're welcome to skip to chapter 3, *What To Expect, The Good, The Bad, and Staying Healthy*. Otherwise, I'll be taking you step-by-step through the process of moving off of your birth control, options that are available if you're struggling to become pregnant, and what health risks you should be aware of that can affect fertility.

Moving off of Hormonal Birth Control

First of all, your body doesn't need to be "cleansed" off birth control. Unlike drugs like sleeping pills and SSRIs (selective serotonin reuptake inhibitors), your body won't go through withdrawal from stopping your birth control, whether you're taking a tablet, are receiving an injection, or are using an intrauterine device (IUD). If you're taking a pill, however, be aware that stopping the pill halfway through the month can lead to menstruation a day or so afterward. This is normal and nothing to worry about, but if you would rather skip that discomfort, stop taking the pill at the start of the new cycle.

A Brief Review of the Menstrual Cycle

The female body naturally produces estrogen and progesterone which are involved with menstruation. Estrogen is the hormone responsible for ovulation, and progesterone is responsible for maintaining pregnancy. During the average menstrual cycle (in the absence of birth control), day 1 - 6 is when menstrual bleeding occurs and the top layer of the endometrium (the layers that make up the womb) is shed from the body. That's why it can be so painful for many girls and women, as an entire layer of the endometrium is stripped and removed.

After this, estrogen levels will gradually increase, causing the endometrium to thicken over time in preparation for a possible pregnancy. Around day 10 - 12, estrogen will rapidly increase, causing a **peak** in concentration, which also stimulates the release of luteinizing hormone (LH) and follicle-stimulating hormone (FSH). This **peak** is important because if there isn't a dramatic enough increase in concentration, ovulation won't take place. Around day 14, ovulation takes place and there is a

24-hour window for fertilization to happen before the egg cell degenerates. Estrogen concentration initially decreases dramatically, after which it becomes a more gradual decrease until the cycle resets. The follicle that had released the egg cell becomes a temporary structure called the corpus luteum, which then begins to produce high levels of progesterone to prepare the endometrium for implantation - the attachment of a fertilized egg cell to the endometrium. Progesterone increases over the next few days and also stimulates an increase in thickness of cervical mucus, to prevent any more sperm from entering. When no fertilization has taken place, the corpus luteum stops secreting progesterone, the structure decays, and the progesterone levels will decrease at about the same rate as they had been produced until the cycle resets. If fertilization did take place, the corpus luteum will remain to continue producing progesterone to maintain the pregnancy, and the remainder of the cycle will not take place.

From this, you can see how important both estrogen and progesterone are for not only *causing* and *maintaining* pregnancy but also for *preventing* pregnancy depending on when they are introduced into the cycle, as well as the concentration of the hormones during the cycle.

Armed with this knowledge, I'll now take you through each contraceptive method and explain how they either mimic or disrupt the natural cycle to prevent pregnancy and how to stop using them.

Pills, patches, and injections

You've probably noticed that there are dozens of different birth control pills available today. The reason for this is that many of them differ in the amount of hormones that are in the formulation. Most of these tablets are made up of a combination of estrogen (or its variant, estradiol) and progesterone (or progestin). There are some formulations that contain only progestin. The combination pills simulate the menstrual cycle in its entirety, without the ovulation part as there is no **peak** in estrogen concentration toward the middle of the cycle. Menstruation still takes place, as the body is fooled into thinking ovulation took place, that the phantom egg cell wasn't fertilized, and the endometrium lining still gets shed. There are, however, options nowadays that completely prevent menstruation as well for convenience. Pills that only contain progestin, fool the body into thinking that you are pregnant, as progesterone is normally only consistently present for pregnancy, so ovulation won't take place and fertilization can't take place.

Why does the pill sometimes "fail"? This could be due to a few reasons. One way to still become pregnant even while on the pill is that accidentally skipping a dose can cause an **estrogen peak**, which causes ovulation. Another way the pill can fail is if the combination you are on is not suited to your body, often because the estradiol concentration is too low. If you're unhappy with your pill, whether it's because of breakthrough bleeding or bad side effects, don't hesitate to speak to your family medicine doctor or OB-GYN to find a solution that works for you.

Birth control patches function in a similar way to the pill, except the hormones get absorbed through your skin instead of through your digestive system.

The injection (Depo-Provera) contains progesterone only and has a longer-lasting effect compared to the pills and patch, as it creates a literal depot of progesterone in the body, which prevents ovulation and prevents the entry of sperm through the cervix.

For pills and patches, it can take 1 - 3 months after stopping to become pregnant, depending on your body and how quickly it starts up its own estrogen production.

After stopping the injection, it can take 10 - 18 months for women to become pregnant, and thus this form of contraception isn't advised if you plan to have a family in the next year or so.

IUD

The IUD is a device inserted within the uterus, that releases levonorgestrel (which works in the same manner as progesterone), which prevents pregnancy by preventing fertilization through thickening of the cervical mucus so that sperm can't gain access, by making the area of the uterus fatal to sperm, and by thinning the endometrium lining.

Ovulation can take place within a month of removing the IUD, however, pregnancy may only happen within 6 months to a year.

Implants

A contraceptive implant is a device that's usually inserted in the upper, non-dominant arm, which gradually releases progestin to prevent ovulation. Like the IUD and injection, it can take a longer period of time to become pregnant after removing the implant.

Vaginal Ring

As the name suggests, this ring-shaped device is inserted inside the vagina and depending on the composition you are using, either releases a combination of progestin and estradiol, or progestin alone, to prevent pregnancy. Most women are able to ovulate again 1 - 3 months after removing the vaginal ring.

Take away

Due to the long-term nature of hormones, it's advised to stop the use of any hormonal contraception a year ahead of when you plan to become pregnant. Working with an OB-GYN or family medical doctor during this process can also help. To prevent any "oopsies" from slipping through, it is advised to switch to a non-hormonal form of contraception (for example condoms) during this period.

It's incredibly important that you see a medical professional if you experience any unusual side effects during the use of hormonal birth control, or after stopping hormonal birth control, particularly headaches, unusual bleeding, light-headedness, and severe mood disturbances.

Struggling to become pregnant

Sometimes it can be a little harder to become pregnant, but you don't have to give up hope! There can be many causes, such as irregular ovulation, structural abnormalities that have to be surgically corrected, polycystic ovary syndrome (PCOS), and more. If you're struggling to become pregnant, consult a family medicine doctor or OB-GYN for advice and assistance for the next step. I will briefly discuss the most common causes with you so that you are prepared going in and know what to expect.

Causes of Fertility Issues

As I mentioned, there can be many causes of fertility problems. It does take two though, so the issue isn't necessarily on the woman's side. The following are just a few well-known causes of fertility problems. There are definitely more but I wanted to touch on just a few.

Fertility risks in women:

- Obesity - Aside from the other health-risk factors, obesity can interfere with fertility because of insulin resistance and hyperinsulinemia (higher than normal levels of insulin in the blood) which causes higher levels of circulating estrogen, and this prevents ovulation. Furthermore, higher levels of adipose tissue (fatty tissue), can disrupt gonadotropin-releasing hormone (GnRH; the hormone released by a part of the brain, called the pituitary gland, that's overall responsible for the reproductive cycle), and prevent the forming of follicles for ovulation.

- Smoking - The chemicals contained in cigarette smoke can cause menopause 1 - 4 years earlier, can increase the risk of miscarriage and decreases fertility due to faster degeneration of follicles.
- Alcohol - Alcohol can disrupt the GnRH system, which further disrupts the release of LH and FSH, directly contributing to infertility as this disrupts the normal hormonal cycle that assists with ovulation and implantation. Additionally, high alcohol use causes oxidative stress, which means less oxygen is available for the reproductive systems to function normally.
- Diabetes - Both Type I and Type II Diabetes mellitus can cause irregularities in the menstrual cycle, which in turn causes issues with ovulation. These issues include infrequent menstruation or even a lack of menstruation. In young women with low BMI scores with Type I Diabetes mellitus, there can be a decrease in GnRH

secretion (and a decrease or lack of ovulation). Type II Diabetes is usually linked with obesity, of which the effect on fertility has been discussed. Menopause may occur earlier. If the diabetes is under control, however, there is evidence of improvement in fertility.

- PCOS - This is one of the more common causes of decreased fertility, as PCOS is defined by abnormal hormone levels in the female reproductive system, and particularly affects the ovaries. Due to hormonal disruption, ovulation may not always take place, menstrual cycles can be irregular and infrequent, or prolonged. There may be an increase in male (androgen) hormones in the body (in the female body, low levels of androgenic hormones are normal), which causes symptoms like more body hair, short temper, and acne. PCOS can also cause the ovaries to be enlarged and surrounded by follicles, which disrupts their function. The symptoms can get worse if you are obese and/or have diabetes.
- Excessive exercise/physical activity - Although inherently not dangerous or harmful, high levels of activity such as that seen in professional athletes can cause temporary infertility. The likely cause of this is the fact that extreme exercise will cause an increase in corticotropin-releasing hormone (CRH), which will disrupt the release of GnRH, thus effectively blocking the

reproductive cycle, as the body is diverting resources toward being active, instead of reproduction. A decrease in physical activity (within reason) usually switches the reproductive cycle back on.

- Endometriosis - A chronic condition where the endometrium lining begins to grow outside of the womb (uterus) itself. The condition is painful, although, 20 - 25% of women are asymptomatic. It's unclear what causes endometriosis as of yet. Laparoscopic surgery is usually used as surgical treatment to remove cysts or to remove excess tissue. This, however, is only temporary and the endometrium lining will outgrow the uterus again. Pain management is used additionally. It's believed that endometriosis affects fertility due to changes in the pelvic anatomy, it may cause disruptions in the normal hormonal cycle, and could cause the fertilized egg to be unable to implant in the uterine wall.
- Fibroids - Fibroids are the most common, benign (not dangerous), tumors that form inside the womb. How this impacts fertility is inconclusive, but it could be due to disruption of implantation of the fertilized egg, they could form a physical barrier and can cause changes in the frequency of contractions in the uterus.
- Other hormonal disruptions - Any condition that can disrupt the reproductive hormones at any point, whether in the brain (GnRH) or within the womb (estrogen,

progesterone, LH, FSH) can cause infertility. There is a large number of conditions known and unknown that can have an effect on the reproductive hormonal system, such as mental health conditions, thyroid complications, certain infections, and more. If your menstrual cycle is abnormal, or ovulation does not take place regardless of everything else being functional, it is up to a medical professional to diagnose your condition and advise you on the best treatment strategies.

- Age - Fertility decreases with age due to many of the body's systems gradually slowing down. Eventually, women reach menopause, where the reproductive cycle stops completely. This occurs between the ages of 40 and 50 for most women. After menopause, a woman can no longer become pregnant.
- Cancer - Various different kinds of cancer can cause physical obstruction and/or scarring, can be the cause for removing the womb (hysterectomy) and other structures important to pregnancy or can decrease or increase the release of hormones that decrease fertility. The different cancer treatments also have a very negative effect on fertility.

Fertility Risks in Men:

- Obesity - Just as in women, obesity can cause infertility in men as it can lead to smaller sperm concentrations, and the sperm become less mobile (the ability for sperm to move efficiently is called sperm motility). One of the possible reasons for this is that obesity leads to oxidative stress, so the cells in the body don't get enough oxygen to function normally, this includes reproductive cells. Another possible reason is an increase in body temperature, as sperm aren't formed and die easily at higher temperatures. Finally, more adipose tissue causes hormonal imbalances, specifically less testosterone in the body and more female hormones, which causes a direct decrease in sperm production.

- Diabetes - Diabetes also causes oxidative stress. Glucose (the main source of energy the body uses and primarily comes from sugars and starches that we eat) is important for sperm production, and in diabetes, the body's ability to metabolize glucose, i.e. to use and store it properly, is disrupted, which can directly lead to less sperm count.
- Prostatitis - The prostate's main function is to produce a fluid that nourishes sperm cells and also makes up a part of semen. Prostatitis is when the prostate is inflamed, either due to an infection, injury, or immune system disorders. Sometimes it can be temporary due to infection and have no long-term consequences, but in chronic cases, it can cause issues in fertility, as well as discomfort and other health issues.
- Urethritis - Urethritis is when the tubes that transport urine from the bladder are inflamed, usually due to infection, but can be due to injury or physical obstruction. The reason why it can cause infertility is that

it can lead to inflammation of the epididymis, where sperm are stored and reach maturity. This can cause a decrease in sperm count, and no sperm in the semen. Obstruction of the tubes and ducts within this system due to inflammation also directly influences the transport of sperm.

- Cryptorchidism - This is a condition where one or both of the testes don't descend, meaning that the testes themselves are still contained within the body itself (the scrotum is a sack that helps the testes to hang outside the body for temperature regulation). Due to the body's warm temperature, the teste(s) can't produce sperm.
- Testicular Torsion - Rarely, the testicles (usually only one testicle) rotate, causing the spermatic cord to twist and prevent blood flow to the testicles. This needs to be surgically corrected. The decreased blood flow causes a decrease in sperm production and overall function of the testes, and possible lesions caused by surgery may also cause infertility. It's not always possible to salvage the testicle, but the odds of success are higher in younger men.
- Cancers - As mentioned with women, different cancers can have various negative impacts on fertility, whether because reproductive structures had to be removed (such as a testis), physical obstruction due to the tumor or scar tissue left from surgical removal, and disruption of the

normal hormone system that causes a disruption in sperm production. Cancer treatments also have a very negative effect on the cells and systems in men.

- Varicocele - A condition where the veins within the scrotum become enlarged, which causes decreased blood flow in the scrotum, and oxygen-poor blood pools within the veins. Poor blood flow means less oxygen to the cells and structures, meaning decreased functioning and decreased sperm production. The pooling of blood also increases temperatures around the testes, which we now well know isn't good for sperm. It is the most common cause of infertility in men, affecting 40% of men who tested for infertility.
- Heart and lung conditions - Aside from all the other issues that come with them, heart conditions like high blood pressure and heart attacks can cause a decrease in fertility, as heart conditions are associated with higher oxidative stress. The same with lung conditions like emphysema. Essentially any condition affects the transport of oxygen through the body, as every cell needs oxygen to function. Oxidative stress means less oxygen, as well as the presence of free-roaming toxins in the blood that can kill cells.
- Genetic disorders - There are many genetic disorders that can cause infertility, whether because of genetic mutations that cause no sperm to be produced, lower numbers of sperm, dysfunctional sperm, or dozens of other dysfunctions.

- Age - As with women, fertility decreases with age, however, men don't stop producing sperm from a certain age. Instead, the contributing factors are usually a decrease in testosterone levels, which decreases testicular function and libido. Additionally, with increased age, there is more risk of other conditions like urinary tract infections, prostatitis, and more trouble achieving an erection, all of which negatively impact fertility.
- Smoking - The effects of smoking on men are more difficult to determine than on women, however, the toxins inhaled through smoking increase oxidative stress, and there is some relation to decreased sperm counts and sperm motility.
- Alcohol - A very recent study found that heavy alcohol usage causes a decrease in sperm concentration, whereas previously it was believed to decrease semen concentration. Other than that, drinking a lot of alcohol also causes oxidative stress, and may also cause sperm DNA fragmentation, meaning that sperm are dysfunctional at a genetic level.
- Injuries and Surgery - Any physical injury, and/or surgery in the scrotum or around any of the structures involved with the male reproductive system, can decrease fertility due to physical obstruction, or lesions that cause a decrease in hormonal secretions.

Fertility Treatment

Don't let the previous sections scare you off, or dishearten you if you recognize one or two of these factors within yourself. Not all of these risk factors are permanent, and there are many treatments available to assist. Whether the treatment is condition-specific, such as managing diabetes with metformin and/or insulin, other treatment options are available that specifically target fertility.

Fertility Treatment for Women

Once you've consulted your OB-GYN or family medicine doctor if you have trouble becoming pregnant, they will likely start by determining the cause, and then prescribe the most suitable treatment option available for you. These include medication, surgery, intrauterine insemination (IUI), and in vitro fertilization (IVF).

Medication:

This list refers to medication that directly affects the reproductive system. Other conditions that can contribute to infertility have their own lists of prescribed drugs to manage them, and will not be discussed here.

- Clomiphene (Clomid): One of the first drugs that were registered to assist with fertility, is clomiphene. It is a selective estrogen receptor modulator (SERM). It works by increasing the amount of GnRH released from the pituitary gland, which increases FSH and LH levels, thus stimulating ovulation. It is particularly prescribed for women who ovulate irregularly, or who don't ovulate at all. The use of clomiphene does increase the chance of twins because it can stimulate multiple follicles instead of just the usual one. The most common side effect of clomiphene is mood swings, and 10% of women may experience hot flashes. Other side effects are very rare and temporary, however, if any visual disturbances (blurry or double vision) are experienced, clomiphene treatment should be stopped immediately.

- Letrozole (Femara): Letrozole is an aromatase inhibitor. Aromatase is an enzyme part of the estrogen production process, and letrozole blocks it from working. The way it stimulates ovulation is as of yet unclear, although it could be via complex feedback mechanisms. It's usually prescribed for women with unexplained infertility, or for women who didn't respond to clomiphene, and is usually used in addition to IUI and IVF.
- Tamoxifen - Like clomiphene, tamoxifen is a SERM, although it has a slightly higher chance of ovulation and pregnancy compared to clomiphene.
- Gonadotropin preparations - These are drugs that mimic the naturally occurring gonadotropins (FSH and LH) and their functioning to induce ovulation.

- Gonadotropin-releasing hormone antagonists - These drugs function by blocking the natural GnRH hormone from working in the brain. This prevents LH from peaking prematurely, as these drugs are usually used alongside IVF.
- Metformin - Metformin is particularly prescribed for women with PCOS who have not responded to clomiphene. Because PCOS causes insulin resistance, metformin counteracts this by increasing the body's sensitivity to insulin and thus can act as an ovulation stimulant. It's the first line of medication prescribed to individuals with Type II Diabetes, and can also improve insulin sensitivity in obese individuals. Women with diabetes will likely already be controlling their condition with prescription medication.

Surgery:

This is normally employed if there are physical obstructions causing infertility or is the primary line of treatment in the case of endometriosis and fibroids.

- Removal of obstructions, scar tissue, and corrective surgery - If there is something physically preventing sperm from accessing the egg cell, or preventing the egg cells from moving through the fallopian tubes, these obstructions can be surgically removed. Similarly, scar tissue, whether from previous surgeries or other injuries, can also cause some obstruction and need to be surgically treated. When there are structural abnormalities, whether due to infection, injury, or inherited reasons, corrective surgery basically "corrects" the structures to help them function in a more normal way.

- Myomectomy - This procedure refers to the removal of uterine fibroids. If fibroids are present, they must be surgically removed, as they do contribute to infertility, as well as to prevent them from becoming malign (cancerous) as time goes on.
- Surgical treatment of endometriosis - This refers to the removal of any endometrial tissue that has spread outside the womb and the removal of any cysts. The removal is done either via excision, i.e. cut out, or via ablation, i.e. destroying the unwanted tissue through freezing, burning, laser, or electricity.
- Laparoscopic ovarian drilling (LOD) - This is a surgical treatment option for women with PCOS. It entails creating three to eight punctures in each ovary with either a laser or via diathermy. Likely the destruction of ovarian follicles causes a decrease in androgen hormone levels, causing FSH levels to rise and restore ovulation.

Assisted Conception:

This refers to treatments that often involve a combination of hormone and drug treatments in addition to the options discussed below.

- Intrauterine insemination (IUI) - Also known as artificial insemination. This line of treatment is usually used in cases of male infertility, endometriosis, and unexplained infertility. It entails artificially inserting sperm into the womb via a thin plastic tube.
- In vitro fertilization (IVF) - IVF is usually preceded by hormonal therapy so that the ovaries produce multiple egg cells. These egg cells are then collected and fertilized with sperm in a laboratory, outside of the body (in vitro), and multiple embryos are then transferred to the mother's womb. Multiple embryos are used, as it increases the odds of implantation as not all embryos survive. This however does also increase the chance of twins or even more babies.

Fertility Treatment for Men

Medication:

- Clomiphene - As discussed above, this works by increasing the amount of GnRH released from the pituitary. What this also does, is increase testosterone levels, which is necessary for sperm production.
- Anastrozole - This drug is also an aromatase inhibitor and prevents testosterone from being converted into estrogen. This leads to higher testosterone levels, meaning improved sperm production, sperm count, and improved sexual drive.

- Human chorionic gonadotropin (hCG) - This is a hormonal treatment that directly stimulates the testes to produce more testosterone, and thus improves sperm production.

Surgery:

- Removal of obstructions, scar tissue, and corrective surgery - Just as with women, removing any blockages, or correcting any abnormal tissue, can improve sperm delivery not only throughout the testes but also to the egg cell.

Lifestyle Changes That Can Improve Fertility

Living as active and healthy a life as possible is always the best and first place to start. Here are some changes you can implement at any point in your life, even if you're not planning on becoming pregnant.

- Maintain a healthy BMI. This is important as obesity increases the risk not only for infertility, but also other conditions that in turn also contribute to infertility, such as diabetes, and heart conditions.
- Exercise regularly, but in moderation. Overdoing it can have the opposite effect.
- Follow a healthy, balanced diet; i.e. stick to foods high in antioxidants, eat leafy greens like broccoli, regularly consume fiber, reduce carbs and sugar, and choose high-fat dairy over low fat.

- Get the right amount of sleep.
- Stay hydrated, drink 8 glasses of water throughout the day.
- Don't smoke.
- Limit alcohol use.
- Limit caffeine intake to a maximum of two cups of coffee per day.
- Maintain healthy iron levels. Don't take iron supplements without a healthcare professional's advice, however.
- Avoid multiple partners and any promiscuous behavior that can increase the risk of contracting sexually transmitted infections (STIs).
- Avoid handling strong toxins like pesticides, and strong cleaning products (as in the industrial kind, your dishwasher soap is safe).
- If you're planning on becoming pregnant within the next year or so, avoid riskier activities that can cause injury, such as extreme sports.
- Men should avoid wearing tight underwear and tight pants.
- Eliminate unnecessary stress.
- Women should take supplements containing folic acid, vitamin D and vitamin B12 when they start trying to conceive.

Surrogacy

Whether you're still struggling to become pregnant, or can't become pregnant yourself for other reasons, surrogacy is always a viable option. Surrogacy entails another woman carrying your baby. There are two kinds of surrogates, a traditional surrogate, and a gestational surrogate.

With a traditional surrogate, the surrogate mother is the biological mother. The male parent's sperm is then artificially inseminated, and the surrogate mother will carry the baby for the couple and hand it over for care once she's given birth.

With a gestational surrogate, IVF is used, where the sperm and egg cells of the parents are fertilized and then implanted in the surrogate mother. So, the baby's parents are the biological parents, the mother just wasn't the one actually pregnant with the baby. With gestational surrogacy, the parents could have also used an egg or sperm donor, or both.

The process of surrogacy differs from state to state, and how involved the surrogate mother is in the baby's life after birth also varies from situation to situation.

Surrogates can be friends or family members, or you can make use of a surrogate agency.

When choosing a surrogate, make sure of the following:

- They are at least 21 years old.
- They've given birth to at least one healthy baby before.

- They don't have a history of mental illness or other serious health issues.
- Sign a contract with them stipulating everyone's role and what happens before, during, and after the pregnancy.

3

What To Expect, The Good, The Bad, and Staying Healthy

Are you pregnant?

One of the first questions you might be asking yourself unless you're reading this after you've already confirmed it is if you're pregnant. Usually, this question pops up when your period is late, or if you're experiencing some of the early symptoms of the first trimester like nausea (what many people call morning sickness), sudden sensitivity to smells, and sore, tender breasts. The only way to be 100% sure is to do a pregnancy test. Doing a pregnancy test after having unprotected sex and missing a period is always advisable. If you and your partner are trying to conceive, naturally you'll want to test for pregnancy.

There are several home pregnancy test kits that you can buy at a pharmacy that test for human chorionic gonadotrophin (hCG) to be present in the urine. Don't rush to the toilet the day after you and your partner tried to conceive, however, you should wait at least 6 - 12 days as that's approximately how long it takes for the fertilized egg to implant in the uterus and start producing hCG. A negative test can be a false negative, particularly if the first test was done very early. Take another test a few days later just to make sure, as chemical pregnancies (see chapter 6 *Complications*) are something that can occur as well. Essentially these are situations where the egg cell was fertilized, the first test may be positive, but the cell didn't implant for some reason, which means no pregnancy will take place. A second positive test is a very sure indication of pregnancy.

Follow the instructions of the pregnancy test exactly, and if you're taking any medication, check that they don't interfere with the result of a pregnancy test either. For the most accurate readings, the tests prefer midstream urine, as that's the most concentrated. Basically, it wants you to pee for a second so that the first diluted urine gets eliminated, then you hold and can put the test or cup for testing in place and release the rest.

Don't let the prices of pregnancy tests fool you, the cheaper tests are as accurate as the more expensive tests. Some of the more expensive tests promise approximations of how much time has passed since ovulation or other nice bonuses, but these readings are less accurate, and it's all up to you what you want from your pregnancy test.

If you're certain you're pregnant, but the store-bought tests keep coming up negative, it's best to consult a medical professional. At the end of the day, the most reliable way is always to have a pregnancy test done by your OB-GYN, family medicine doctor, or at a fertility clinic around the time that you're supposed to have your next period and missed it.

When you're seeing a healthcare practitioner to confirm your pregnancy, they will order a blood test and a urine test. The blood test can determine 100% if you're pregnant as this determines the exact amount of hCG present in the body. The extra urine test is just to cover all the bases. A physical exam may be conducted but isn't a requirement to confirm pregnancy when a blood test is done. A physical exam entails looking for signs of pregnancy like an increase in the size of the uterus, changes in the color of your vagina and cervix, and changes in the texture of the cervix.

Congratulations, you're pregnant!

From here on out, I'm assuming you've tested positive for pregnancy, and will now guide you through the screening tests, trimesters, what you might experience, and offer advice on what to eat and drink, what to avoid, and what medications are safe.

Your First Consultation and Prenatal Care

If your first consultation is after you've already tested pregnant, that's no problem at all. Not all pregnancies are planned, and even if yours is planned, most women who go for consultations before confirmation of pregnancy are those who have tried to become pregnant but are struggling and looking for advice.

I've already discussed how to pick your healthcare professional in chapter 1, *Choosing Your Healthcare Provider*, and so we will now go over what your consultations will look like if you've tested pregnant.

Your First Consultation

This appointment will likely be the longest, as this is usually the appointment when blood tests are done (or at least ordered) not only to confirm your pregnancy but also to check other important factors in the blood:

- Hemoglobin and iron levels: Hemoglobin is the protein that enables red blood cells to transport oxygen and carbon dioxide throughout the body. Iron is a mineral essential to forming hemoglobin. If hemoglobin and iron levels are low, you could be anemic, meaning that the different cells that make up your body aren't receiving enough oxygen.
- Your blood type and Rh factor status: It's important for healthcare practitioners to know your blood type in case

of emergencies where blood infusions are necessary. The Rh factor is an inheritable trait that determines what type of protein is found at the surface of your red blood cells. Every person either has a positive Rh factor or a negative Rh factor. Although it doesn't make any difference if the Rh factor of an adult is positive or negative for everyday functioning, it does come into play when blood infusions are necessary, and when the factors of the biological mother and biological father differ. More on the hemolytic disease of the newborn under chapter 4, *Delivery Time*.

- Detection of infections: To ensure your and the baby's safety, you're going to be tested for the possible presence of infections like hepatitis B.

A urine test may also be done, to additionally confirm pregnancy as mentioned before, but also to check for the possible presence of urinary tract infections (UTIs).

Your practitioner will help you calculate your estimated due date (EDD), which is generally calculated as 40 weeks. Some pregnancies may last 39 weeks, or 41 weeks, which still falls within the normal range. The 40 weeks are calculated from the first day of your last menstrual period, as this is the most accurate way. How the calculation works, is you subtract 3 months (12 weeks) from the first day of your last period, then add 7 days. Fortunately, nowadays there are apps that can help you with the calculation. If you have irregular periods, this method likely won't be as accurate. No need to worry though, as an early ultrasound (done during a later consultation) can give you a more accurate timeframe from your practitioner.

During your first consultation, your practitioner will ask about your medical history. Your medical history includes the following:

- Immunizations you've had and when (if you don't have records of your childhood immunizations, this can be determined through a blood test as well).
- Operations you've had, no matter how small or inconsequential you might think it is.
- Illnesses you've had in the past, for example if you've had mumps or meningitis.
- If you have any chronic illnesses you're aware of, for example diabetes.
- If you're diagnosed with a mental health condition, for example anxiety and or depression.
- If you're using any medication at present. Mention everything that you're using, even if it isn't a medication for a chronic condition. Even if you don't think it's important to mention, mention it anyway.
- If there's any family history of certain conditions. For example, if your father has high blood pressure, or your grandma on your mother's side had breast cancer. Even

if you don't have the condition, if a family member has it, there's a greater chance for you to develop it due to similar genes. This includes mental health conditions, not just "physical" conditions.

- Alcohol, smoke, and/or other substance use. It's important to be 100% honest, as this information is incredibly important to your and the baby's health. Many people who do smoke, or use recreational drugs, may feel too guilty or embarrassed to share this with their practitioner, usually out of fear of being judged, or fear of being admitted. In cases of pregnancy, however, it's very important to remember that not only your health is at stake here, and a good healthcare provider isn't supposed to judge you or do anything against your will.
- How much caffeine you consume on average. This includes coffee, tea, and energy drinks.
- What your sexual history and lifestyle are, i.e. if you've had multiple sexual partners and in what time period, if and what birth control was used, etc.
- Your practitioner will measure your weight and height and calculate your BMI to determine your health.

Your practitioner may also conduct a breast and pelvic exam during this consultation to cover all the bases and determine your overall health. Other physical examinations can include measuring your blood pressure, heartbeat, and lungs.

Your healthcare provider will likely discuss factors of your lifestyle with you that weren't covered by your medical history and may suggest changes for a healthy pregnancy. These lifestyle factors include your diet, how active you are, and what type of work you do, i.e. something that involves a lot of sitting like a desk job, or something that involves more physical labor, like nursing, as well as the workplace environment. Other factors can also include how susceptible you are to stress and the stresses you're currently under.

You will very likely be prescribed supplements, particularly folic acid and calcium. Folic acid (or vitamin B9) is incredibly important for DNA and RNA synthesis (which is how cells and proteins in the body are formed), and doubly so during pregnancy. Birth defects due to folic acid deficiency are easily preventable by taking supplements. Furthermore, pregnant women are highly recommended to take calcium supplements, as your body is providing the growing baby with all its calcium requirements during pregnancy. If there isn't enough calcium in your body, calcium will be taken from your bones to be used elsewhere, causing your bones to weaken and increasing the risk of osteoporosis and other bone diseases. Taking calcium supplements will ensure that you and the baby get enough calcium for both of you to function.

Lastly, your practitioner will ask about any symptoms you're currently experiencing and may prescribe medication to help to manage the worst. Don't put on a brave face, if you have pain or nausea or anything bothering you, discuss it. The right healthcare provider will never judge you or belittle what you're experiencing.

Prenatal Consultations and Screening

The testing doesn't stop with the first consultation. Throughout your pregnancy tests will be done to ensure your and the baby's health. Another exciting part about this is determining the baby's sex and sometimes revealing that there's more than one baby partying it up in the womb.

Genetic Screening

Genetic screening involves tests to determine if you and/or your partner carry any genes that can carry over genetic conditions to the baby. It's highly advised to do this *before* becoming pregnant, as it can inform many decisions regarding your pregnancy. These tests screen for Down Syndrome and spina bifida in particular, but can include hemophilia and sickle cell anemia. Fortunately, many conditions are only inheritable if *both* parents carry the relevant genes. In some cases, only one parent has to carry the gene, such as hemophilia only being transferable from the mother's side if the baby is male. If only one partner has an inheritable condition, such as an autoimmune disease, there is a 50% chance of the baby inheriting it, depending on which parent's genes they inherit.

First Trimester (Week 1 - Week 12)

For many women, this first trimester can come as a bit of a shock to the system. Even if there's no bump (yet) to give yourself away, your body is undergoing a lot of changes. Your hormones are going crazy, your favorite food is suddenly the most unappealing thing in the world, and why on earth are you craving ice cream so badly? The first trimester is not just morning sickness and cravings, however.

Over the next few weeks, your baby will develop from a fertilized egg cell (called a zygote), and go through various developmental stages throughout this trimester that doesn't necessarily look very human at first, but by week 18 in the next trimester, what started out as a little bean will very nearly resemble the baby they'll eventually grow into.

Symptoms to Expect

- <u>Tender, larger breasts:</u> Even though some women wouldn't mind a free breast enlargement, this one is only temporary and can come with discomfort. Your breasts can start increasing in size weeks after conception. The reason for this is simple, your body is preparing to feed the coming baby. Other than the size difference, the hormonal changes can cause your areolas and nipples to darken; the idea is to make it an easier target for a hungry baby to find. This darkening may go away after birth, or may only turn a slightly lighter shade. Light-skinned ladies will also notice the veins and arteries under the skin more properly, as more blood carrying important nutrients is being pumped into your breasts. These hormonal and size changes are what cause sore, tender feelings. Hot or cold compresses (whichever you prefer) can alleviate the pain, as well as a more comfortable bra without an underwire. Don't worry though, the worst of it will pass by month 3 or 4. Something to keep in mind is that not enough breast support throughout your pregnancy can lead to more saggy breasts afterward, but you can go easier during the first trimester.

- "Morning" Sickness: This is something of a misnomer and should be renamed All-the-time sickness, as most women who experience nausea during pregnancy, don't necessarily experience it during mornings alone. This refers to nausea with vomiting, and nausea without vomiting. Sometimes there doesn't even have to be a trigger and you'll just wake up with an unbearable feeling of nausea. Scents and smells that once were pretty normal, or even nice, may now suddenly yank at your gag reflex. If you can't keep your food down, there's no need to worry about your baby's needs just yet, as they're still just a tiny bundle of cells at this point and don't need that much fuel to keep growing.
- The exact reason why 75% of pregnant women experience nausea during pregnancy isn't quite clear. It

could be due to the dramatic hormonal changes, it could be the increased sensitivity to smells and food, or it can be due to the relaxation of the sphincters and muscles of your gastrointestinal tract. Regardless of whether you only occasionally feel nauseous, or are nauseous all the time, it's often one of the worst symptoms for women to go through. For most women, fortunately, it only lasts for about 6 - 12 weeks, basically half of the first trimester, and will begin to calm down once they transition into the second trimester.

- Some tips for managing nausea include: eat smaller meals more frequently, eat blander foods like toast and crackers (the BRAT diet, which stands for Bananas, Rice, Applesauce, and Toast, is commonly prescribed for upset tummies as they are relatively bland, easy foods to eat, and will give you most of the necessary nutrients to get past this hurdle), stay hydrated (preferably with water, and if you're vomiting a lot, try some rehydration preparations that contain electrolytes), ginger - whether ginger candies, ginger infused tea (decaf of course), or ginger cookies, this root has proven over and over again to be quite effective at managing nausea. If a certain food or supplement makes you nauseous (iron supplements can be a culprit), avoid the foods that trigger you, and talk to your practitioner about possible alternatives to get those important supplements inside of you. Injections aren't everyone's cup of tea, but if you can't keep a tablet down, this might be the better option in the short term. And of course, you're welcome to talk to your practitioner about medication to manage your nausea if it's unbearable. The currently accepted treatment worldwide is ondansetron, and although there is some research that reports risks, there isn't enough evidence yet to indicate whether it's truly dangerous or not. Other alternatives to ondansetron are anti-histamines like cyclizine (often taken for car sickness), and prochlorperazine.

- <u>Frequent Urination:</u> Something that's unavoidable about pregnancy, is that you're going to need the loo more than ever before, and this might continue even after the baby is born. Those hormones are the culprit again, as they'll be increasing the blood flow in your body, meaning your kidneys will be working more, which means more regular restroom breaks. On top of this, your uterus will slowly start to grow and will literally start pressing on your bladder, triggering the need to go more frequently. The second trimester will bring a little bit of relief, as the uterus will move up into the abdominal space. To reduce the number of trips to the bathroom, once you've finished urinating, try squeezing to see if there's anything left in your bladder. Leaning forward can also help to empty the tank more efficiently. Don't think this is a reason to cut back on fluids however, you should always stay hydrated, as water keeps your kidneys safe and functioning by "oiling the machine", additionally you'll have a better chance of preventing UTIs if you stay hydrated and go when nature calls.

- Headaches: There are literally dozens of things that can trigger headaches, even without pregnancy hormones thrown in to complicate things. Your hormones can cause headaches by making you more congested (and sinus headaches are some of the worst), headaches caused by fatigue, overheating, and their close cousin, dehydration. Low blood sugar is also something to look out for. And unfortunately, now you're very limited on what you're allowed to use to tame these headaches. Acetaminophen-containing medication, like Tylenol, is now your go-to. Just don't exceed 2400mg of acetaminophen daily. If you're headaches still don't go away, or you need to take medication for headaches for more than 3 days straight, you should see a doctor. Before rushing to the pharmacy, however, see if drinking a glass of water and eating a fruit or a small meal doesn't send the headache packing.
- Cravings and aversions: This is not cliché. Due to the first trimester being the most chaotic when it comes to the hormone department, you might out of nowhere experience cravings for food you have never really eaten

before, and will find yourself almost gagging at things you used to love. The cravings are usually just one or two food items, ranging from sweet to salty. Common cravings include ice cream, chocolate, fries, and fruit. On the exact opposite end of this spectrum, you'll suddenly find the thought of chicken (one of the most common aversions), or veggies of all kinds absolutely repulsive. A misconception is that this is your body's way of "telling you what you need", but just as hormones can send mixed signals and cause havoc during puberty, in the same way, hormones can cause confusing feelings and messages to be sent during pregnancy. Cravings are usually only an issue when it leads to unhealthy eating habits. No need to cut out the comfort foods completely, but try to find healthier substitutes that can pacify the cravings to keep you and your baby healthy, for example try roasted potatoes instead of McDonald's fries, or some sweet fruit instead of an entire tub of ice cream. If you find yourself craving non-food (this is called pica), report it to your practitioner as many of these non-foods can be dangerous if the temptation gets too strong.

- Fatigue: Do your knees feel weak, and your arms heavy? Does walking from the bedroom to the kitchen make you feel like you just ran a marathon? Do you feel exhausted and ready for bed, but it's only 11 am? Well, your body *is* creating a little human, and although the little baby is little more than a pea, there's still a lot of work going into building the placenta, making sure your little pea gets enough nutrients and oxygen, on top of all the other changes to prepare your body for the rest of the pregnancy and caring for a baby after birth. Pregnancy is the perfect excuse to take lots of breaks, to be kind to yourself, and to be pampered by others. If your body needs to go to bed early, then go to bed early. Take time at the end of the day to fully relax with a nice book or movie. Healthy snacking is encouraged to keep those energy levels up, and although it might not feel like it, a walk or slow jog can also help.

- <u>Heartburn:</u> Unfortunately, you'll be very likely to experience heartburn while you're pregnant, even if you were lucky enough to dodge it before becoming pregnant. The gastroesophageal valve, between your esophagus and your stomach, will relax a little while you're pregnant, meaning there's a greater chance of reflux (the stomach contents pushing up into the esophagus, causing the horrible burning sensation), or for stomach acids to leak through, especially while lying down. You can prevent this by avoiding foods that can trigger heartburn, such as spicy foods, citrus, and fried food.
- <u>Constipation:</u> Yup, another reason to spend longer periods on the toilet. This is unfortunately another fairly

common symptom caused by high levels of progesterone in your body. The motility of your digestive tract slows down a little, which means that something of a traffic jam can occur on the way out. Iron supplements don't exactly help either (on top of coloring your poop dark). Ways to combat constipation before switching to medication are by drinking lots of fluids, high-fiber foods, some exercise, and prunes. There's a reason the elderly drink prune juice. If your body remains stubborn, however, there are suppositories as well as oral meds that can help to bring some relief, but make sure to discuss first with your practitioner or a pharmacist what's safe to use during pregnancy.

- Excess Saliva: Pairing this with nausea can be a very unpleasant experience for many pregnant women. Your body might start producing more saliva than normal, making for some awkward conversations and a more active gag reflex. Fortunately, chewing sugarless gum and using minty dental products can help to dry things out a bit.
- Metallic Taste: This is a rarer symptom and doesn't always get mentioned, but some women may experience an odd, metallic taste in their mouth as if they'd accidentally bit their tongue. Just as your sense of smell becomes oversensitive during pregnancy, so does your sense of taste (the two are closely linked after all). You

can relieve this annoyance by brushing your tongue, rinsing your mouth with a salty solution (about a teaspoon of salt in 8 ounces or 240 ml of water), or by eating some citrusy fruits (if they don't cause you heartburn), or sucking on some citrus candy.

- Emotional: Frankly, you'll be all over the place. From crying over a pair of cute baby booties to wanting to hit your partner for an innocent comment. Get used to wearing your heart on your sleeve and having a harder time watching those emotional movies you might have loved. Your hormones are going crazy, and so will your emotions. Stress and worry are also normal, your body is the host of a brand-new little human! If it gets too difficult to distract yourself or find ways to calm down and relax, get help from loved ones and/or a professional. There's no need to suffer in silence.
- Spotting: So, you thought you'd be spared from your period for the next 9 months? You will be, don't worry, but you might experience spotting, i.e. a little bit of blood early in your pregnancy. No need to panic. Sometimes during implantation, when the embryo makes itself nice and cozy in the uterine wall, it can cause a little bit of bleeding. During pregnancy, the walls of your cervix also become a bit more tender and can easily be irritated by friction, such as during sex or physical exams, which can cause a little bleeding.

- Bloating and Gas: Again, due to progesterone's effects on the digestive tract, this can cause uncomfortable gases to build up and create unpleasant pressure in your tummy area. Don't be embarrassed by the little toots that escape either, it's healthier to get rid of that gas than to keep it in, and it's a normal part of pregnancy.

When To Call a Professional

Naturally, your body is going through all sorts of changes causing all sorts of sensations that can be worrisome. Most of these are normal and will pass after a few months. However, if you experience any of the following, it's safest to contact a healthcare professional as soon as possible:

- Heavy vaginal bleeding, bleeding with severe cramps or pain in the lower abdomen.
- Severe, persistent pain or cramps in the lower or upper abdomen even without bleeding.
- Decreased urination or even a complete lack thereof.
- Painful, burning urination.
- Blood in your urine.
- A fever over 101°F or 38°C.
- Any visual disturbances, such as blurry vision, double vision, seeing spots or any trouble seeing normally.
- Sudden onset of puffiness around the face, eyes, and hands along with a bad headache and trouble seeing.

- Severe headaches, and headaches that last longer than 2 - 3 hours.
- Feel constantly faint or dizzy.
- Chills with a fever, but no other symptoms.
- Severe nausea and vomiting.
- Frequent diarrhea, especially if it has a slimy appearance
- Itching all over, with or without yellowing skin and eyes (jaundice), pale stool, or dark urine.
- If you get the feeling that you need to. Sometimes you might not be experiencing any serious symptoms, but your gut is telling you something's wrong. It's better to be safe than sorry.

Other Things to Keep in Mind

As I've already mentioned several times, there are a lot of hormonal changes happening in your body, that can lead to some other unexpected changes that aren't necessarily always good or bad. Some other things that could happen during pregnancy are:

- Hair changes. The hormones during pregnancy can either make your hair bouncier and shinier than ever before or make it go limp. Moreover, you might be growing extra hair in all the usual places as you're turning into a Carebear. Fortunately, the extra hair can be safely removed through all the usual methods, just keep in mind that your skin is likely to be more sensitive.

It's also better to avoid any chemical or heat-based treatment of your hair, as overheating a pregnant body is generally a bad idea, and coloring uses chemicals that may be absorbed through the skin, and you may breathe in the fumes during the process. Color treatments that don't directly touch or affect the scalp, like a lovely ombre, could be safer, but be sure to check in with your healthcare practitioner first.

- Acne-like you're back in high school. They don't really show this one on tv or in the movies, but pregnant moms can develop this annoying skin problem due to more oily skin (thank you hormones). You can still use facial cleansers, scrubs, and the like, or even go for a facial, as long as you avoid retinoids, beta-hydroxy acid (BHA), and salicylic acid. Accutane is a serious no-go. Always make sure that a product was tested to be safe during pregnancy before using it. Remember, your skin is an organ that absorbs things that can end up in your bloodstream. Laser treatments and facial peels are also better left off until after your baby is born, even if only to protect your oversensitive skin.
- Avoid the heat. This includes overly hot baths, making the bedroom too warm for bed, and even saunas. And no tanning beds, ever. If you're going through most of your pregnancy during the winter months, keep your feet warm with some nice, thick socks and cuddle up with

your partner, or invest in some fluffy, fleece blankets. Increasing your body temperature too high can harm your developing baby by turning your womb into an unpleasant kind of oven.

- Try using cleaning products that don't contain strong chemicals; organic products are usually the safer route. Avoid pesticides, whether bug spray or during gardening, at all costs. These chemicals can be absorbed through your skin and are highly toxic.
- No need to avoid nuts if you're not allergic. Studies show that women who withhold eating nuts during pregnancy are more likely to have children with nut allergies. This way you can start developing their immune system ahead of time. The same goes for other common food allergies. As long as you're not allergic and the food isn't to be avoided by a pregnant mom, you're welcome to drink that glass of milk along with your breakfast of scrambled eggs.
- No need to evict the cats. Yes, cats and cat litter are carriers of toxoplasmosis, which is harmful to babies, but if you're a longtime cat owner, chances are you've developed a natural immunity that will be transferred to your baby. Additionally, indoor cats are highly unlikely to carry diseases compared to toms wandering the neighborhood. If you're unsure if you have toxoplasmosis immunity, a simple blood test can

determine it. If you don't have immunity, have your cats tested, and if they tested positive for toxoplasmosis, have someone look after them for the next 6 or so weeks. If they don't have toxoplasmosis, keep them inside and don't let them hunt or eat any raw meat. And perhaps ask your partner, family member, or friend to help with the litter box, just to be safe.

- Make sure your tap water is safe, not only for drinking but for brushing your teeth and washing fruits and vegetables.
- Make sure there are no traces of lead in the paint on your walls, or if you've inherited some old furniture, like the cot your grandpa made.

Checkups During the First Trimester

I'm assuming you've at least had your very first checkup with your chosen healthcare practitioner as discussed under *Your First Consultation and Prenatal Care,* and are now going in for routine checkups as scheduled.

In your second month of pregnancy, approximately weeks 5 - 8, your checkup will include weight and blood pressure measurements, urine tests for sugar and protein in your urine, examinations for swelling around your ankles or hands as well as for varicose veins, and you can raise any concerns you may have or ask any questions.

In month 3, approximately weeks 9 - 13, you'll be entering your second trimester towards the end. Near the end of week 9, you can go for NIPT if your practitioner thinks it's necessary, your health insurance covers it, and you want to go for it. Otherwise, your very first ultrasound will take place somewhere from week 10 to 12. Although your baby is still teeny tiny, your practitioner will look for their heartbeat. In addition, they will continue to measure your weight and blood pressure, examine you for any signs of swelling or varicose veins, and will determine the size of your uterus by feeling from the outside, as well as the height of the top of your uterus (called the fundus). Any questions or issues you have can of course be brought up.

If diagnostic tests are necessary, you'll be going for CVS at 10 - 13 weeks based on the results of NIPT and/or NT.

Baby's Development

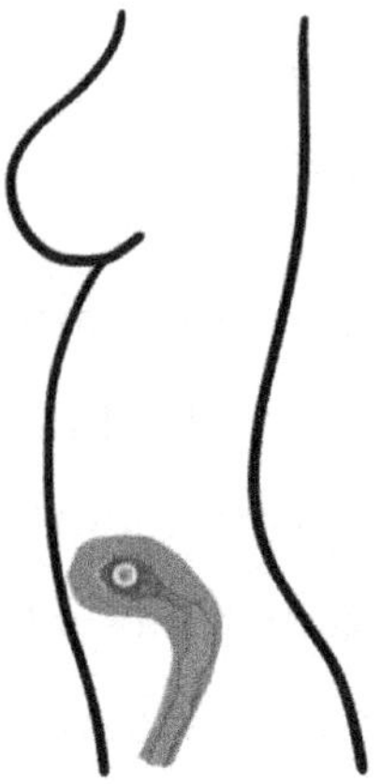
WEEK 0-6

Week 1: This week begins on the first day of your last menstrual period because there's no way to accurately determine exactly when the sperm fertilizes the egg, the exception being IVF of course. So, no baby just yet.

Week 2: As ovulation takes place this week in preparation for The Big Meeting between your egg cell and the lucky sperm that gets to fertilize it, there's still no baby yet. The uterus is thickening, preparing the nest for a possible new baby.

Week 3: Your egg cell and sperm cell met, joined in fertilization, and have now become a zygote. This little blob of a cell will start dividing and dividing over and over again, steadily growing in size, until it becomes a grape-like structure of cells called a blastocyst. The blastocyst will now get into the fallopian tube and start to slide down to the uterus.

Week 4: The blastocyst has now become an embryo, a teeny tiny vaguely baby-shaped bundle of cells, that begins to implant into the uterus lining. The cells that make up the embryo will now divide into equal halves, one half forming the placenta that will be your baby's bed and breakfast and source of oxygen for the duration of their stay, while the other half makes up the baby. Not unlike a bird's egg, an amniotic sac and a yolk sac are forming as well, and the three cell layers of the embryo are starting to specialize. The yolk sac will eventually become part of the digestive tract. The three layers are the endoderm, which will eventually become the liver, lungs, and digestive system; the mesoderm, which will eventually become the bones, heart, kidneys, and genitalia; and the ectoderm, which will become the skin, hair, eyes, and nervous system.

Week 5: In just a month, the bundle of cells has grown to the size of a sunflower seed, and your baby will look a bit like a cute little tadpole. Their heart and the neural tube will start to develop this week, and you might actually see their heart beating on the first ultrasound. This early on, the little heart only consists of 2 chambers called heart tubes, and the neural tube is still open.

Week 6: This week the baby's lungs, kidneys, and liver will start to develop. Some of their face will also start to develop, including what will become the eyes and ears, a little nub that will become a nose, the cheeks, chin, and jaws.

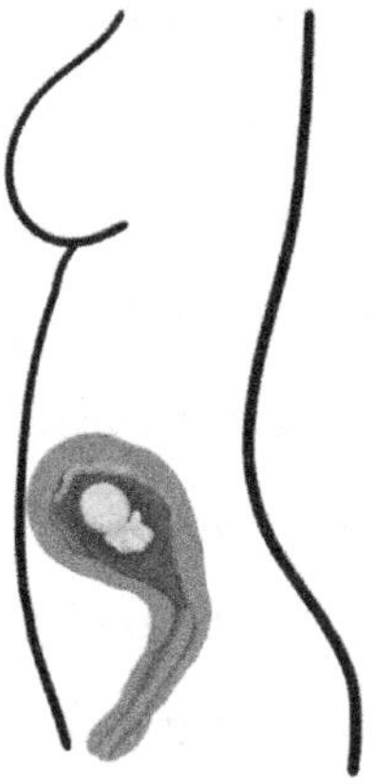

WEEK 7-11

Week 7: Your baby is now roughly the size of a marble. They're beginning to sprout stumps that will become arms and legs, with hands and feet. Their mouth and tongue are also developing, and their kidneys are fully formed by now. On top of that, a lot of the growth is focused on creating thousands of brain cells.

Week 8: By now the baby is looking more like a human baby instead of a tadpole, and its limbs, nose, mouth, and eyelids are continuing to develop. They'll also start moving around this point; tiny little motions that you won't be able to feel. At week 6, their heart rate was about 110 beats per minute, which escalated to 150 - 170 beats per minute in week 8.

Week 9: The baby is now the size of a grape and is beginning to develop muscles. It won't be long until you'll start feeling the baby kick and move about.

Week 10: Your baby is now officially no longer an embryo, and is now a fetus! They'll have grown an extra half-inch, have fully functional kidneys and stomach, have developed elbows, and bones and cartilage will form. Baby boys' testes will already start producing testosterone.

Week 11: Little baby's fingers and toes are separated by now and will begin to grow nails within the coming weeks. Hair follicles are developing, the ears, nose, and nostrils are nearly complete, they have a palate and tongue, and little girls will start to develop ovaries. Your baby will no longer be curled up as much either and is starting to stretch out a little bit.

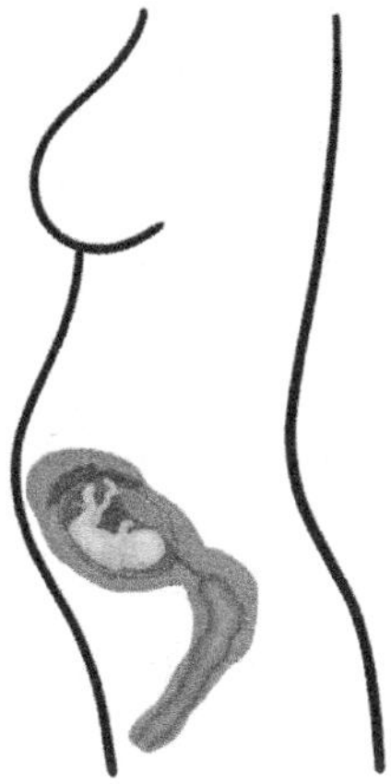
WEEK 11-14

Week 12: Most of the essential systems are now fully formed, such as the immune system, hormonal glands and systems, and gastrointestinal system; they just need to do a bit more growing. The baby is now about 2 inches long, which is double the size it started as this month, and now very nearly resembles the baby they'll be by week 40 in miniature.

Second Trimester (Week 13 - Week 26)

The initial hormonal turmoil usually begins to calm down as you enter your second trimester, meaning the horrible nausea is likely to fade away within the next week or two, as well as the breast tenderness and need to pee all the time. With the second-trimester things tend to mellow out a bit more, as the hormones are settling into their groove and the baby isn't big enough yet to push around and cause discomfort. You can also expect your baby bump this trimester and start taking pregnancy progression pics!

Symptoms to Expect

- Growing Breasts: Yes, your breasts will probably continue to grow for the duration of your pregnancy. Hopefully, the soreness and tenderness are gone by now or will be gone soon, and this is a good time to invest in some comfortable and supportive bras, either with wide straps or sports bras.
- Baby Bump: Although subtle at first, your belly is expanding, subtle enough that one day you'll realize with a surprise that a little bump popped out of nowhere. Some women already started to show in their first trimester; this could be due to bloating, or some weight gain. Nothing to worry about if you're showing your bump at week 6 or week 16. Every woman's body is different, and although there are urban myths about how a woman is carrying and what it means, nothing is supported by scientific evidence. As long as your practitioner confirms that the baby is healthy, and you're happy and healthy, that's really all that matters.

- Braxton Hicks Contractions: These can be scary at first, as your uterus might just start contracting slightly. These contractions aren't true contractions, however, they're not very strong and your baby isn't announcing that they're on the way. The exact reason for why these contractions occur is uncertain, but triggers have been identified, namely if you have a full bladder, have just had sex, are dehydrated, did some exercise, or are highly stressed. The only time to become concerned is if the contractions become incredibly painful, they become longer and longer, and if the frequency between contractions increases.
- Increased or Decreased Sexual Drive: For some women, the hormonal surge also means that they're nearly constantly in the mood. This is thanks to increased blood flow to the pelvic area and genitalia, making them more sensitive and tingly. On the opposite end of the spectrum, the over-sensitization and symptoms like nausea completely kill the mood. Both sides of the libido coin are normal, and you should respect your body's needs and boundaries. If you're not up to cuddling, communicate that to your partner and explain what you're going through. If you're rearing to hop into bed, but your partner's not up for it for their own reasons, you should also respect their needs and boundaries. Pregnancy is a weird and wonderful experience, and

even though you and your body are bearing the physical and emotional brunt of it, it does have an effect on your loved ones as well.

- Stretch Marks and Pigmentation Changes: The only true way of preventing stretch marks is through good skin elasticity. Stretch marks are scar-like marks that vary from silvery-white, to purplish-pink, to reddish-brown, and are formed due to micro-tears in the skin due to excessive stretching, or sudden expansion. You can avoid stretch marks by inheriting good genes (so not something you can exactly control), exercising regularly, eating healthy, and keeping weight gain gradual (and healthy). As of yet, moisturizers and oils don't prevent stretch marks or can make them disappear, but that shouldn't discourage you from keeping your skin healthy and moisturized with pregnancy-safe products.
- Hormonal changes may also cause some pigmentation on your skin, due to an increase in melanin, the cell responsible for the color of your skin and hair. Tanned-looking patches, called melasma, may appear on your skin and are likely to disappear after your baby's birth. Sun exposure is also more likely to trigger melasma, or even aggravate it. Limiting time spent in the sun is a general rule of thumb, and you should always apply sunscreen when going out, even if it's cloudy.

- Sensitive Gums and Other Dental Issues: Increased sensitivity also applies to your gums, and not just your skin, sense of smell, or well, everything. Your normal flossing and brushing routine may cause bleeding, so a gentler routine and softer brush are recommended. Rinsing your mouth with salt water, or a mild mouthwash can help prevent infection and soothe inflamed gums. If you're vomiting frequently, the high acidity could affect your tooth enamel, so good dental hygiene should be maintained. It's also best to leave most dental treatments until after the baby's born and your mouth isn't as sensitive anymore, emergencies being the exception of course. Just be sure to notify the dental practitioner that you are pregnant so that they only use products that are safe for pregnancy.
- Varicose Veins and Spider Veins: First of all, varicose veins and spider veins aren't the same things. Spider veins are red or purplish lines that fan out from a central point, almost like a spiderweb or a squashed spider's legs. They're usually harmless and it's only the appearance that some find off-putting. Spider veins are caused by inflammation and stress on the tiny blood vessels in your body, which can make them visibly stand out. Genetic predisposition also plays a role in whether or not you'll develop them. Regular movement and exercise that promotes blood flow can help with

prevention. There is a chance for your spider veins to disappear after pregnancy, and if not, can be treated by a dermatologist.

- Varicose veins, on the other hand, are when the veins close to the surface of the skin become enlarged, and/or twisted, usually on the legs. This isn't limited to pregnancy alone. Anyone who leads a more sedentary life is vulnerable to developing varicose veins, as are people who do most of their work standing (such as teachers, nurses, and pharmacists). In pregnancy, as with spider veins, the increased blood flow puts pressure on the veins of your body. This is often painful and can cause swelling of the ankles, muscle cramps, burning or throbbing in the affected leg, eczema, and scar-like marks. To prevent varicose veins, it's recommended to move around, exercise, and take breaks from sitting every now and then to get the blood moving. Compression socks are also a viable option if you don't have the luxury to move around a lot. Otherwise, varicose veins can be treated through laser or sclerotherapy but this is only to be done after your pregnancy.
- Vaginal Discharge: You might notice a thin, clear, or whitish discharge in your underwear. This is normal. It's called leukorrhea and is meant to protect the cervix and exit route clean of infection, as well as to maintain a

healthy flora balance. It can be annoying to clean out of your underwear, and tampons are not advised in this situation. It's also supposed to only have a mild smell, so if you notice any changes in the smell or color, or experience any kind of burning or itching in the downstairs department, you should consult your practitioner. Other than that, don't try to "clean" down there, as this is the body's way of making sure it's clean. Douches, feminine wipes, and soaps can disturb the pH and natural bacteria in the area, which can lead to infections that are more uncomfortable to deal with than the mildly annoying discharge you were dealing with initially.

- <u>Dizziness:</u> Surprise, surprise, hormonal changes can cause feelings of dizziness, and changes in blood flow and blood pressure in different parts of the body can lead to bouts of dizziness and feeling faint, especially when suddenly moving. Low blood sugar can also contribute to faint and dizzy feelings. If the dizziness persists and doesn't go away, consult a practitioner in case you have some kind of insufficiency contributing to this.
- <u>Nasal Problems:</u> As I mentioned under headaches, pregnancy tends to make your nose more congested, and on top of that the increased blood flow and inflammation of your nasal membranes can cause them to bleed easier. To prevent frequent nosebleeds and unnecessary

congestion, try keeping your environment humid with a humidifier, staying hydrated, and clearing your clogged passages with a saline solution. Decongestant nasal sprays are only to be used if your practitioner says they're safe, and long-term use can paradoxically cause your nose to become clogged all over. And yes, your congested schnozz may mean that you'll suddenly become a snorer and feel like you constantly have hay fever.

- <u>Backache:</u> This is one of the most frequent complaints of pregnant ladies, and you can often see someone with back pain walking with their hands supporting their lower back, and belly out. Not only is your body carrying additional weight in a part of the body that's throwing it a bit out of balance, but your pelvic joints are also loosening up. Switch up standing and sitting, as doing either for too long can start to put a strain on your back. This will also be a good reason to invest in a desk chair that provides good support for your back and neck, with cushioned armrests. A footrest to slightly elevate your feet is also a good idea. Don't get into heavy weight lifting around this time either, and if you already were, it's better to switch to lighter weights for a while and make sure that anything heavy is lifted slowly.
- <u>Changes in Blood Pressure:</u> Small changes in your blood pressure are normal. You might have slightly elevated

blood pressure due to the increased blood flow throughout your body. During the second trimester, your blood pressure is likely to drop a bit due to how much work is going into making a baby, and then will pick up again around the third trimester. Blood pressure readings become more concerning when your systolic is around 140 and up, and your diastolic is around 90 and up. In cases like this, your practitioner will closely monitor your blood pressure to eliminate the white coat effect (a phenomenon where patients only have high blood pressure when examined by a healthcare professional). A 24-hour blood pressure monitor will be the best way to determine your overall blood pressure on an average day. If you have high blood pressure readings along with swelling of the face, hands, and ankles, and/or severe headaches, this could be an indication of preeclampsia.

- <u>Sugar in Your Urine:</u> If you weren't diabetic before you became pregnant, this doesn't mean that you are now. Some women's bodies slip up a bit in the process of ensuring that their baby gets all the glucose they need. Essentially, their bodies want to make sure there's enough glucose in the bloodstream for both mom and baby, and insulin is responsible for regulating the amount of free-roaming glucose, so they slightly inhibit its function. In cases where they do the job too well, some excess glucose that neither mom nor baby need ends up floating around, and so gets dumped into the urine to be removed. Diabetic women should also note that during pregnancy that they're urine will show elevated levels of glucose during pregnancy.

- <u>Out of Breath All the Time:</u> It's those hormones again. Your respiratory system is stimulated to take deeper breaths more frequently, which can make you feel out of breath, and so any slight increase in activity can make feel like running a marathon. The muscles of your respiratory are also more relaxed, creating the sensation that you're not quite filling your lungs. Another cause would be your baby growing, which in turn makes your uterus expand pushing it up into your abdomen when pushes on your lungs. Your baby is perfectly fine in the midst of all this. If you're experiencing chest pains, panic, or find your lips and fingertips turning blueish, it's best to see a practitioner a.s.a.p.
- <u>Hemorrhoids:</u> An unfortunate experience you might have during pregnancy due to the increased blood flow and pressure downstairs, is hemorrhoids. These are actually normal vascular structures inside your rectum, that can become sore and inflamed. If they're internal, you're not likely to feel any pain, but going Number 2 or anal sex can cause them to bleed. External hemorrhoids can look like varicose veins that are often itchy, painful,

or even cause a burning sensation. There are topical hemorrhoid creams available for treatment, you can take a bath in Epsom salts (just make sure the water isn't too hot), many women find that wipes containing witch hazel help, apply an ice pack to the area for at least 15 minutes every day, and avoid sitting for long periods of time. To prevent hemorrhoids, make sure to eat a high fiber diet, go to the toilet when you need to go no questions asked, don't strain too much while on the toilet, and as always, exercise.

- Initial Fatigue: Don't worry, toward week 18 you should feel a change in your energy levels and will likely spend your second semester feeling more energetic.
- Pregnancy Brain: If you were usually the one who was on top of things, remembered every appointment, and always knew where everything was, this might be frustrating to experience. Your thoughts might be drifting mid-conversation, or you'll wander into the kitchen and not remember why you're there, or you're forgetting birthdays and leaving your car keys in the fridge. You're not going senile, so-called pregnancy brain is very common. You have a lot on your plate, after all, your body is creating a brand new little human, your hormones are all over the place, and there's just so much to do and prepare! So be kind and patient with yourself, and if a relative or friend becomes impatient with you, ask them to be patient as well.

- Popped Out Belly Button: Toward the end of the second trimester, your belly button might become an "outy" due to the pressure behind it. It will return to normal, so no need to worry. It's essentially a scar of where your umbilical cord used to be when you were just a baby in your own mother's belly.
- More of the Same: Many of the symptoms from your first trimester will likely persist into the second, and even the third. If you were lucky to dodge them in the first trimester, you might have them in one of the others. These include heartburn, constipation, bloating and gas, and headaches.

Checkups During the Second Trimester

Either at the end of your first trimester or at the start of your second (between weeks 11 and 14) your practitioner might request a combined test if they feel it's necessary.

For your first checkup this trimester, between weeks 14 - 17, you can expect more weight and blood pressure measuring, examinations for swelling and varicose veins, and urine tests. Your practitioner will also continue to monitor your baby's heartbeat, the size of your uterus, and the height of the fundus, and will discuss the symptoms you've been experiencing. As always, bring up any questions or concerns.

Between weeks 14 and 22, you will undergo quad screening or integrated screening.

If amniocentesis is necessary, it'll take place between week 16 and week 20.

In the fifth month, weeks 18 - 22, you can expect more of the same from your checkup; weight, blood pressure, swelling, varicose veins, urine tests, fetal heartbeat, size and shape of the uterus, fundus height, and any symptoms you may be experiencing. You will also receive a level 2 ultrasound, where you'll finally be able to see your baby and perhaps even see its sex.

In the sixth month, (weeks 23 - 27), you will receive the same standard checkups as in month five, but this time there will be an additional glucose test.

After week 24, AFI (Amniotic Fluid Index) is measured. AFI is a standardized test used to measure the amount of amniotic fluid present in the amniotic sac. Too little or too much amniotic fluid is a complication (see Oligohydramnios and Polyhydramnios).

Baby's Development

<u>Week 13</u>: As you enter the second trimester, your baby is nearly 3 inches long, and the intestines that have been developing in their umbilical cord are beginning to transition into their body.

<u>Week 14</u>: Here's when babies will begin to grow in size and length at their own pace, which will also be the case once they're born. The overall development, however, remains the same for

all babies. Your baby might start to grow hair on top of its head, and its eyebrows will start to come in. Your baby will also grow a little furry coat to keep them warm called lanugo, which most babies shed once they start to accumulate fat.

Week 15: Your baby is now 4 inches long, and their eyes and ears are moving into their correct positions; the ears to the sides of the head, and the eyes to the front of the face. Your baby is also much more mobile now, as they'll start to wiggle and kick, suck on their thumb, and will practice motions similar to breathing and swallowing for when they'll actually need it. The baby is still too small for you to feel these motions just yet.

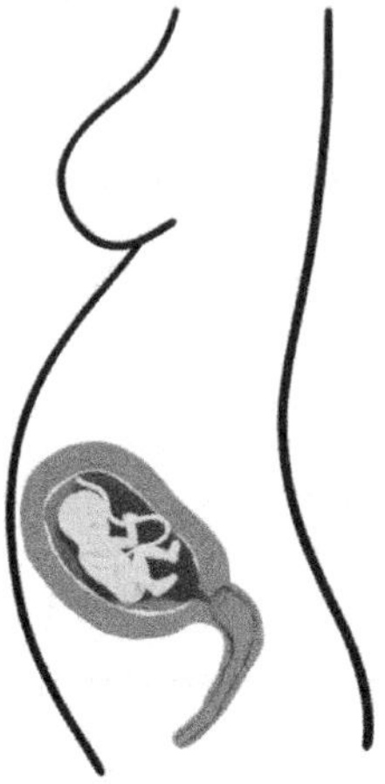

WEEK 15-18

Week 16: Baby's muscles have developed enough for them to straighten out more, and their face is now that of the tiny baby you will meet in a few weeks, now with eyelashes! Their eyes have also developed considerably, although their eyelids are still sealed, their eyes are capable of movement, and can somewhat detect light.

Week 17: At 5 inches, your baby is picking up the pace in the growth department. They're still practicing swallowing and suckling, and are starting to develop some baby fat on their little body. Their skin is still somewhat translucent though. The autonomic part of your baby's brain has also taken over regulating their pulse, which is now about 140 - 150 bpm.

Week 18: You might start to feel some of your baby's little movements and kicking as they're doing acrobatics in there. They now have their own unique sets of fingerprints, truly setting your baby apart. They've also started to learn how to yawn, and can even get the hiccups!

Week 19: Your baby now ways approximately a whopping half a pound, and is about 6 inches long. To prevent your baby from turning into a wrinkly prune during their holiday in the amniotic fluid, a white, greasy layer called vernix caseosa is now coating them all over. A little before their time comes to emerge into the world, they'll shed their greasy coat. Some premature babies are born still wearing their cheese-like coating.

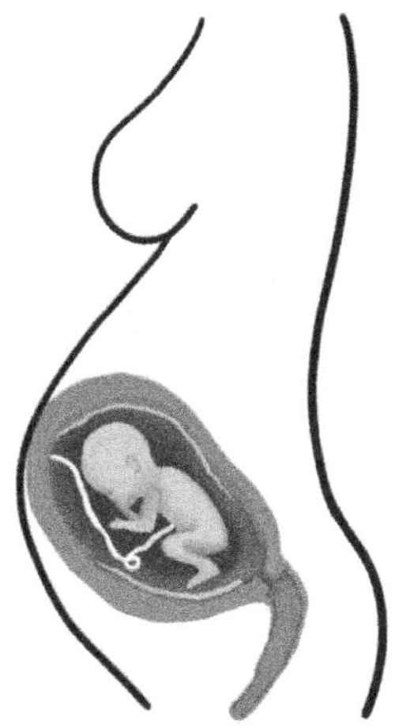

WEEK 19-22

Week 20: Time to find out what your baby's sex is (unless you want to keep it a surprise?)! This week, your baby is big enough for an ultrasound to pick up their genitalia if they're not hiding them with a foot or are being shy. A baby boy's testicles will begin their journey down from the abdomen, where they will eventually enter the scrotum which is still in development. A baby girl has fully developed ovaries that are storing around 7 million baby egg cells.

Week 21: Your baby is now a little longer than a soccer ball in diameter, from head to rump that is. The neurons in their brain are now connected to the appropriate functions, and the relevant cartilage structures are becoming bone, giving your baby more control over their movements. Their arms and legs are also in the right positions and proportions now, which means you're very likely feeling them move around now.

Week 22: They've hit the 1-pound mark! Your baby is also now around 11 inches long. They're practicing their grip by holding onto their umbilical cord, which will give them surprising strength once they're out in the world. They can now also hear all the sounds your body's making, your intestines working away, the rhythm of your heartbeat, the rush of your blood, and of course your voice. They can also hear some sounds from outside, albeit muffled versions. Their eyelids are still sealed, but their eyes can detect the difference between light and dark.

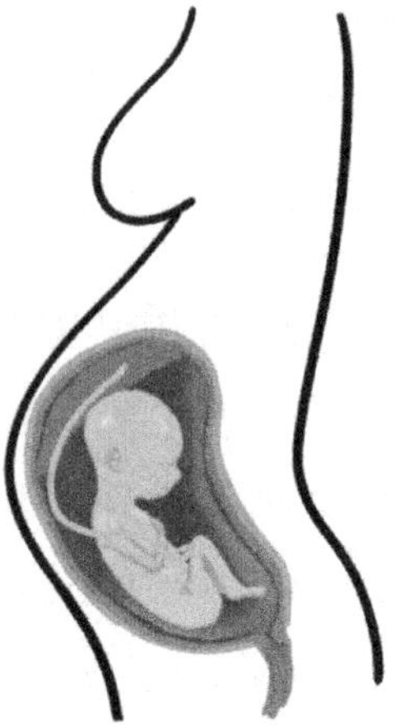

WEEK 23-26

Week 23: Your baby is still semi-transparent due to the lack of baby fat, so you can see the red of their veins and arteries, and can see their bones underneath the skin, which they still need to grow into somewhat. They'll fill out soon enough though.

Week 24: As predicted, your baby is gaining about 6 ounces a week in baby fat, as well as organs and bones that are continuing to develop. Their head is now practically fully developed, except what hair they might have doesn't have any pigment yet, so their hair will appear white outside the womb.

Week 25: This week your baby's just over a foot in length! Their little lungs are starting the first steps to developing what will be their respiratory system; air sacks with capillaries (called alveoli) are beginning to form inside the lungs, in fact, capillaries are forming everywhere under the skin. They're also beginning to develop surfactant, a compound on the surface of alveoli to keep them from collapsing by lowering surface tension. Little baby is still a while away from breathing on their own. You might start to feel them getting hiccups however as they begin to practice breathing-like motions, as well as due to their vocal cords now being fully developed.

Week 26: You are now nearing the end of the second trimester and are heading for the third, and final few weeks of being a living bed and breakfast. Your baby now weighs a stunning 2 pounds! On top of that, their eyelids have been unfused and their eyes can start to open! However, just like kittens and puppies who open their eyes for the first time, your baby's irises don't have a definite color yet due to the lack of pigmentation.

That's why many newborns have that dark blue-grey eye color until their true color inherited from mom or dad develops. This is also not a good time to attend events with bright flashing lights, as your baby will notice them and you might even feel them get startled by sudden bright light or loud noises.

Third Trimester

After the relative calm of the second trimester, things begin to ramp up again in the third. Your belly will start to become uncomfortably big as baby takes up more and more space. They might also be keeping you up at night with their antics of training for the circus, or you're lying awake because you're just uncomfortable and feeling too hot. Your back is likely to hurt more as your baby is packing the pounds and you need to carry them around everywhere you go. This is the final stretch though, so hang in there! In just 12 or 13 weeks or 3 months, you'll be holding that little baby in your arms!

Symptoms to Expect

- <u>Fatigue, the Sequel:</u> Your energy levels may have improved during the second trimester, so it's understandably a bummer when the fatigue hits again. The reasons are pretty obvious, as you're carrying a substantial weight around your middle wherever you go, and a 24-hour workout will tire anyone out. Plus, your baby is growing faster than ever before, which means your body is putting even more energy into readying your little angel for the day when they can finally meet you. If you've been overdoing the nursery prepping and baby planning, you should take a break. All of these little things add up to cost you even more energy.

- Swollen Ankles: Are your feet killing you and are unable to fit in your favorite Nike sneakers? This is because of edema. Due to the hormones and increased fluids in your body, you're very likely to become a little squishier in places where some of that excess fluid accumulates. This could be worsened by sitting or standing for too long, so the same rules go as for varicose veins. You can also elevate your legs to help out your circulatory system to move some of that fluid around, and don't be embarrassed by wearing your comfiest slippers, or whichever shoes work best for you.
- Rashes and Skin Bumps: Even though most rashes are harmless, you should always let your practitioner examine them just in case. Among these strange skin situations is something called pruritic urticarial papules and plaques (or PUPP if you want to save your breath). These are annoying little bumps that usually form around the abdominal area, but can also appear on the arms, thighs, and backside. PUPP usually disappears

after birth, but your practitioner will likely prescribe a topical antihistamine to help deal with it until then.

- Sciatica: Because your baby is getting a little big and is beginning to get into position for birth, they might push up against your sciatic nerve in your lower spine, which will cause pain or numbness down your lower back and one of your legs. Hopefully, your baby will switch positions to relieve some of that pressure, but if not, sciatica can continue until birth, and perhaps even a little afterward. If baby isn't being cooperative, you can sit or lie down to relieve some of the pressure; when lying down, avoid the affected side. A heating pad or soaking in a warm bath (not too warm) can also help, as well as the right exercises. You're also welcome to ask for advice regarding non-medicinal treatment, such as a massage or seeing a chiropractor.
- Restless Legs Syndrome: Another reason that might be keeping you up all night. Essentially whenever you're not on the move, like lying in bed to fall asleep, your legs will start feeling achy, itchy, tingly, or even like they're burning, making it impossible to drift to sleep. Unfortunately, medical science doesn't quite know what causes restless legs syndrome (yet), and although there are medications available, they're not safe to use during pregnancy. Some ways you can hopefully prevent these at home include exercise, but not before going to bed, wearing compression socks to bed, identifying triggers like something in your diet, checking your iron levels,

and cold packs or soaking your legs in cold water before bed.

- Clumsiness: Pregnancy can make you more prone to spilling things, tripping up, and generally feeling a bit like a flailing muppet. This is partially due to your looser joints and the shift in your center of gravity due to your growing belly. If you do fall during one of these bouts of clumsiness, you can always speak to your practitioner to make sure everything is okay. The amniotic fluid is a very good protection system however and will keep your baby safe from most mild bumps and falls. It's probably best to leave activities that require more coordination for after your baby's birth.
- Fever Dreams Without the Fever: Noticing your dreams getting stranger and more real? Do they feel like the insane trips of a fever dream, except you're healthy? Once again, we can thank your hormones, your overheating body, and just about everything going on around your pregnancy. Your pregnancy is likely weighing heavily on both your conscious and subconscious, and understandably so, so your dreams might live out your dearest wishes and worst fears around your baby. These are perfectly normal and not indicative of anything wrong with you. Having a nightmare about giving birth to twenty babies and struggling all night to keep track of them doesn't mean you'll suddenly actually give birth to twenty babies, or

that you're a bad mother. There's not much you can do to stop these dreams from happening, except for trying to cool down your bedroom a little to keep your hot body from inducing the weirdness. No guarantees though.

- Aching Ribs: Did I mention your joints are loosening? That includes the joints in your ribs. There can be inflammation of the cartilage attached to your ribs, and of course, all the pressure doesn't help. Support bands can help with some of that painful pressure, and now is the time to avoid any heavy lifting. Your baby's kicking won't help either, and you can gently nudge them to move by bouncing on a pregnancy ball or by doing some pelvic tilts.
- Morning Sickness Returns: Thankfully not as common as nausea experienced during the first trimester, some expecting women do experience nausea again in their third trimester. Once again, it's due to hormones, but now there's also a baby pushing up against your intestines and possibly pushing your food back up as well.
- "I pee when I…": Whether a sneeze, a cough, or laughing at a funny cat video, you might notice your bladder slipping more. Well, you do have little feet tap-dancing away on top of your bladder, so it doesn't take much for the pressure to get too much and a little pee may come out.

- Weepy Breasts: Some women experience their breasts leaking in their final month, or even during the eighth month. This isn't milk, however, so if your breasts are still dry it's not because they're not producing milk. This is a substance called colostrum, some called it "pre-milk". It's essential for any newborn baby to get colostrum in, as it contains important antibodies and proteins to give your baby the jumpstart they need for their new life. If you're leaking a bit before birth, don't worry, there will be enough for your baby once the time comes as you're constantly producing it. If the leakiness becomes too much, you can wear nursing pads to keep your bra and shirt dry.
- More of the Same: As I mentioned in the second trimester, many symptoms will continue up until D-Day (Delivery Day). As before, these include vaginal discharge, constipation, heartburn, headaches, dizziness, nasal congestion, sore legs, hemorrhoids, varicose veins, backache, itchy skin, stretch marks, shortness of breath, more frequent and intense Braxton Hicks contractions, and sensitive gums.

Checkups During the Third Trimester:

During your seventh month, weeks 27 - 31, your practitioner will conduct the same tests and examinations as before, will determine the position and size of your baby by feeling from the outside, do a blood test for anemia, and will give you the Tdap vaccine. The Tdap vaccine is a whooping cough vaccine to protect your baby from it. It's perfectly safe during pregnancy, you won't become sick from it, and since your baby can't be vaccinated while in the womb, this is the best way to protect them from the outside world. You may also schedule a 3D or 4D ultrasound of your baby to get an even better view of them, although these are only done when medically necessary and is only done by skilled, trained professionals. Don't worry, in just a few weeks you can look at your baby as much as you want and spam your social media with pictures of them! If your Rh factor is negative, you will also receive an injection of RhoGAM around week 27.

More of the same tests and examinations occur in month eight, weeks 32 - 35, and sometime between week 35 and week 37, you'll be going for your Group B strep culture. Group B Streptococcus (GBS) is a bacteria that is found on the perineum of about 20 - 30% of women. GBS infection does not usually cause problems in women before pregnancy however, it can cause serious illness in mothers during pregnancy. GBS also causes chorioamnionitis which is a severe infection of the placental tissues. GBS is the most common life-threatening infection in newborns, aside from pneumonia and meningitis. Newborn babies contract the infection during pregnancy or from the mother's genital tract during labor and delivery. If the lab test is positive, it's important to reduce the risk of transmission with the use of antibiotic treatment given to mom while in labor. Babies whose mothers receive antibiotic treatment for positive GBS are 20 times less likely to develop the disease than those without treatment.

In addition to the standard tests and examinations, your practitioner will also examine your cervix and its lining for any thinning (effacement), and to see if any dilation is starting. During this consultation, you should also receive a labor or delivery protocol from your practitioner to know what to do when the big day dawns. This will be based on decisions you and your practitioner have come to together based on your personal preferences, your health, and the baby's health. This will be discussed more in chapter 4, *Delivery Time.*

Baby's Development

Week 27: Guess who now weighs 2 pounds! Your baby also has more tastebuds than they'll ever have postpartum, meaning that they can in fact taste everything you're eating in the amniotic fluid. This could explain why your little one will have a sweet tooth later on, or perhaps prefer savory snacks. Spicy food might even make your baby hiccup, even though you shouldn't really be eating spicy food. But who knows, maybe your baby likes it?

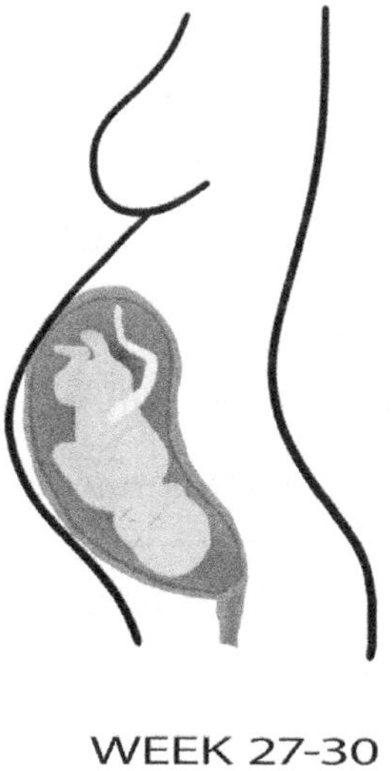

WEEK 27-30

Week 28: Your baby is starting to learn the essential skill of playing peekaboo. Yes, they're starting to blink! Even more amazing, there is evidence that your baby is likely dreaming when taking a nap. What could they be dreaming about? Maybe that song you hummed while doing the dishes while they're doing some kickboxing. It's a pity they don't remember when they're old enough to tell us!

Week 29: Your baby is now training to become a heavyweight champ and is approaching 3 pounds, which will continue to increase until the very end. With them filling out more, your womb is becoming a little small, so you'll definitely feel it when they twist around and do their daily exercise routine.

Week 30: This week, as your baby's body continues to grow exponentially, so is their brain. Humans have the most complex neural systems of all living creatures, so to catch up, your baby's brain is starting to resemble the more wrinkly shapes we associate with it. Their big brain can now take on even more responsibilities, like thermoregulation, which means their furry coat is starting to shed.

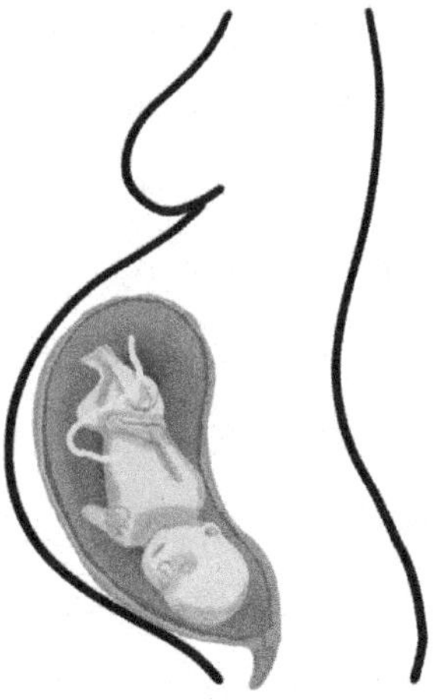

WEEK 31-34

Week 31: Even though your baby still has a short way to go in the weight department, they're very close to their birth length now. This can vary from baby to baby but is usually a little above or below 16 inches. Some women give birth to little giants, others give birth to delicate little dolls, and it's all down to genetics and some other factors. As long as your baby's healthy, size doesn't matter. Your baby's brain is also even better than before and has started up some basic processes. With this extra processing power going on, your baby will also take longer naps.

Week 32: With their baby fat more developed and spread out under the skin, your baby is no longer see-through. And not only is your baby growing physically but so are their skills. This last stretch is a training montage worthy of Rocky as they're perfecting their flailing, gripping, breathing (well, an approximation of breathing), suckling, and swallowing.

Week 33: Your baby is now gaining about half a pound a week, so you know whom to blame for the readings on your scale! The amniotic fluid has now reached max capacity, which also means those cute sensations of your baby's kicks will now become a little more uncomfortable and will likely even keep you up at night. Additionally, your baby's immune system is beginning to develop as antibodies are transferred from your body to them. This is crucial, as the outside world is filled with bugs that can cause all sorts of infections, and this precious little one needs all the protection they can get.

Week 34: If you're expecting a little boy, their testicles will now start their descent. A very small percentage of baby boys are born with undescended testicles, but this usually resolves itself within a few weeks. Your baby's nails are now also fully grown out and will continue to grow rapidly from here on.

Week 35: You're not the only one getting ready for the final stages of this journey. Baby is starting to flip over if they're not already head-down and bottom-up. The safest and most comfortable position for a baby to be born is head-first, facing the rear (cephalic occiput anterior). Some babies are born "sunny-side-up", facing the belly, (cephalic occiput posterior), which can make for a longer, more painful birth (more on complications regarding the baby's position in chapter 6, *Complications*). Your baby's head is getting pretty big now with all that brain development going on, so the easier it is for that big brain to fit through the exit, the better. Fortunately, a baby's skull is specially designed to help them to squeeze through the vaginal canal. Their skull isn't one complete structure just yet and is made up of different regions connected by six structures called fontanelles, making the skull more malleable. The skull regions will start to fuse gradually after birth, with the posterior fontanelle closing by the time the baby is eight weeks old. The rest will be fused by the time your little one is two-years-old.

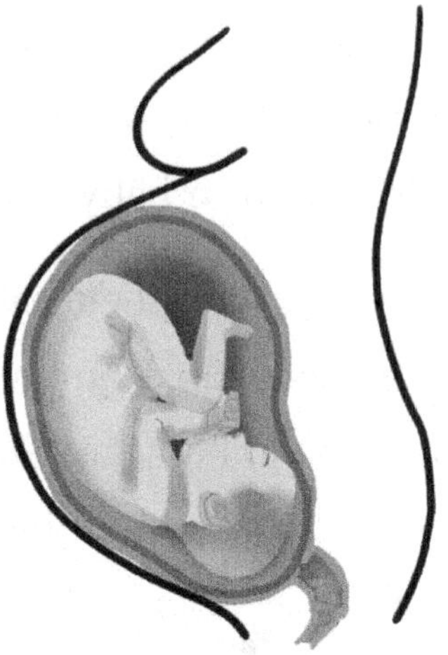

WEEK 35-40

Week 36: Entering the final month, your baby weighs around 6 pounds, and all its systems are developed and ready for life outside the womb.

Week 37: Any birth from this week on is considered full term. If your baby is still happily snuggled away inside, they'll be practicing all their essential baby skills, including cuteness as they continue to pad out their baby fat.

Week 38: Your baby is just about ready to be delivered! This week they'll be shedding the last of their lanugo and vernix, and weigh approximately 7 pounds (give or take).

Week 39: Baby's head is likely in your pelvis, and you might be feeling impatient and like this pregnancy has been going on forever! Just a little while longer.

Week 40: The day first-time moms have waited for. Most likely you have made it to this date, and quite possibly you may have a few more days to go. Don't let this get you down. There is no way but out! You have to birth your baby! You will not be pregnant forever. The two of you made it and have most likely formed a unique bond. Do your best to take a much-needed and necessary nap. Take it easy and don't stress too much. I know, easier said than done, but trust me on this. Pamper yourself, you have a lot of work ahead of you! Delivery, and taking care of your newborn will be discussed shortly, so stay tuned!

Week 41 - 42? Is your baby a little too attached to their cozy room in the womb? There's still no need to worry, although you're probably more than ready to have your baby in your arms by now. Your practitioner won't let the pregnancy go beyond 42 weeks. Your baby might have some dryer skin when they're born, but this is only temporary and will soon be replaced by that infamously soft baby skin. They'll also have slightly longer hair and nails (although some babies come out with a full head of curls at week 40).

You should be feeling your baby move daily. Obviously, they move less as they get bigger because there is less room to wiggle. However, always be vigilant about feeling your baby move. If you feel like you have had no fetal activity recently, you should have a snack or some juice and lay down on your side and do kick counts. Kick counts are basically 10 movements within two hours. If you lay on your side and you feel your baby kick and punch and roll 10 times in the first 10 to 15 minutes, you're done. If you don't feel 10 movements and it has been two hours, call your provider and head to the hospital for an NST (non-stress test).

An NST is an evaluation of fetal well-being using an electronic fetal monitor to monitor fetal heart rate. Other reasons for NST are if the mother is overdue, there's a history of gestational diabetes, diabetes mellitus, preeclampsia, fetal growth problems, expecting multiple babies, abnormal AFI, or a history of intrauterine fetal demise. There are many other reasons for your midwife or doctor to order an NST, but these are just some of the most common reasons.

4

Delivery Time

No one knows how their birth experience will pan out, even if you've already had children. No labor and delivery experience is exactly the same as another. Some labors are over within a few hours while others can take days, but it usually takes 12 - 24 hours for first-time moms. Labor usually shortens for subsequent births.

Knowing the stages of labor and roughly what to expect can help you plan and decide, as well as ease any worries and anxieties you may have. Don't get too attached to your idea of the perfect delivery though; we sometimes see moms cling to a plan in their head, putting unnecessary psychological stress on themselves, which can make it more difficult when the actual day comes. This can also lead to unnecessary feelings of guilt and failure over things beyond their control when this should be a joyous time in their lives.

I'm not going to lie, some women are *adamant* about how they want their labor and delivery to pan out, complete with a laminated step-by-step birth plan. In my experience, these are usually the moms who end up with every intervention done to them from a medical standpoint, and then a C-section. I am probably exaggerating just a bit, but you get the picture. That doesn't mean you shouldn't plan for vaginal delivery though! Just keep in mind the end goal: Healthy Mama and Healthy Baby.

There are no prizes or trophies for having a vaginal delivery. You don't get a special reward for an unmedicated vaginal delivery. Someone isn't a "better mom" for choosing "natural" over having an epidural or needing a C-section. Everyone has the right to choose, and your baby's health and safety are what come first and should always be the determining factor. Sometimes I try to make light when a mom is saddened at having to take a trip to the OR. "It's ok, I had a C-section, and my son still graduated from Cal Poly!" It is usually followed by a chuckle from everyone in the room. There is such a bad stigma on Cesarean Sections. Is surgery the optimal delivery route? No. But most likely if you are needing one, or choosing to have one, it is for a very good reason. In some cases, it would be detrimental to baby's health if mom doesn't have a C-section. So why would you take the chance if that was the case? Just food for thought.

Educate yourself (as you're doing now) on what to expect, familiarize yourself with all the little contingencies that determine which options are viable and safe, and consult your practitioner for advice! This way, your baby's birth will be a wonderful success regardless of how they were born.

Relaxation is by far the most critical skill in mastering labor and delivery unmedicated (if unmedicated delivery is your choice). Relaxation techniques should be practiced early on to release your tense and tight muscles so that your body can remain open and relaxed in the face of labor and delivery. I suggest researching muscle relaxation exercises, visualization techniques, and calming music.

Hopefully, by now you do have a midwife, physician, or some healthcare provider that you trust and are comfortable with. With all my years of experience as a labor nurse, I can't tell you how many times patients didn't trust their practitioner's advice and care. If you don't feel like you can trust your practitioner for whatever reason, then they're not the practitioner for you. In any case, it's our job as nurses to advocate for you, assist you, and care for you and your baby. Our primary goal is your and your baby's well-being, so trust that our guidance is in your best interest.

We as nurses would like you to know that we love what we do. There is nothing more wonderful than the privilege to share in the experience of a new life and assist parents in this joyous and momentous new chapter. Never in my 25 years, at any of the four hospitals that I've worked at, has a decision been made to make the hospital more money. So, trust me on this, we have all the necessary skills, training, and experience to give you the best possible outcome. We truly are not going to do more interventions than we need/have to.

Birthing Baggage

Planning on having the baby at a hospital or birthing center? Whether you have an idea of your due date, have a scheduled induction, or scheduled C-section, you'll need some things with you. Even if you plan on home delivery, it's wise to keep some things packed nearer to the time just in case.

Packing for a visit to the hospital isn't exactly going on vacation though, and it can be overwhelming to decide what to take and what to leave. No worries, over the decades, mothers have compiled lists of essentials and nice-to-haves based on personal experience.

You can pack your bag weeks in advance if that's what your personality is inclined to do, but you can usually start packing around week 36. Some women do end up packing the day before or once they enter the first phase of labor.

Essential Items:

These are non-negotiable; ask your partner, a friend, or a family member to help double-check that these are packed.

- A form of identification, whether ID or driver's license.
- Your insurance card if you have one.
- The name and contact information of your midwife/OB-GYN/family doctor.
- Documentation that your hospital or birthing center of choice needs. Pre-registration usually happens at most hospitals now.
- Cellphone, charger, and multiplug outlet.
- A cord blood kit if you plan on banking your baby's cord blood.
- Infant car seat (to be left in the car until day of discharge).

Personal Items:

Technically, these are also essential for comfort and hygiene, but in emergencies, the above-mentioned items are the most important. Here are personal items that are a must.

- Toothbrush and toothpaste.
- Deodorant.
- Hair ties (if your hair is long enough).
- Soap, shampoo, and body lotion if you prefer to use your own.
- Glasses - if you normally wear contact lenses, switch to the glasses for ease and comfort.

Clothes

You'll be changing a few times, even if you're not staying for a few days, so a change of clothes or two is generally a good idea.

Bodily fluids are likely to be involved, so keep that in mind when choosing what to take.

- Comfortable and loose nightgown or pajamas suitable for IVs and easy access for breastfeeding (if you wish to not wear a hospital gown).
- Light bathrobe (check to see if your delivering hospital gives them out).
- One or two comfortable outfits, like loose-fitting sweats.
- Multiple pairs of postpartum underwear (although most birthing centers provide disposable ones).
- A few pairs of comfortable nursing bras and nursing pads.
- A set of clothes to take baby home in.
- A receiving blanket and heavier blanket for baby.

Nice to Haves

Although not lifesaving, these items are highly recommended to make your trip to the hospital as comfortable as possible.

- Makeup.
- Sugarless candies and approved snacks.
- Your own pillow.
- A camera if your phone won't do the job.
- Earbuds to listen to music or watch videos in privacy on your phone.
- Eye mask and ear plugs.
- Lotion or oil for massages.

- A book, magazine, e-reader, or tablet (and this book if you want!) A laptop with movies installed. These are important if you are having an induction, as you can usually plan on nothing happening for the first several hours.

Rh factor and Hemolytic Disease of the Newborn

Under *Your First Consultation and Prenatal Care,* I explained what the Rh factor is. In many cases of pregnancy, Rh incompatibility occurs. This isn't really an issue during pregnancy itself but can be a problem once the baby is born.

Essentially what happens, is if the mother is Rh negative (her blood cells lack the factor) and the baby inherited the Rh positive factor from their biological father, the mother's body will see the baby's blood cells as foreign invaders, and will release antibodies to deal with the imagined threat. This only happens once the baby's blood comes into contact with the mother's blood, which is why the greatest risk is during the birth itself. Rh positive moms have nothing to worry about.

Hemolytic disease of the newborn (HDN) and jaundice are conditions that can afflict the newborn baby if the mother's immune system attacked them. This causes anemia and an increase in immature red cells (reticulocytosis), which increases the risk of the baby getting sick and even dying.

To prevent HDN or reduce the occurrence of jaundice, mothers' Rh factors are determined early on (usually during the first consultation), and if there is Rh incompatibility, the mother will receive an injection called RhoGAM, which is similar to a vaccine, at the start of her third trimester (usually week 27). RhoGAM contains an Rh-immune globulin that prevents the mother's body from forming antibodies against the baby's blood cells. A second injection is given 72 hours after the baby's birth if the baby is tested to be Rh-positive.

In emergencies, blood transfusion can be done to mask the baby's blood from the mother's antibodies.

Vaginal Delivery and Labor

This is a natural process made up of three stages and is usually only experienced by mothers opting for vaginal delivery. The first stage is your body preparing for delivery, in other words, the labor part of labor. This includes the phases of early (latent) labor, active labor, and transitional labor. The second stage is the actual birth of your baby. The final stage is delivering the placenta.

Stage One, Phase One: Early (Latent) Labor

For the most part, this is the longest phase of labor and is usually (thankfully) the least intense. Signs of early labor would be cervical dilation, effacement (cervix thinning out), and contractions that get stronger progressively over time. Your cervix will dilate to 4 - 6 cm over this period. Sometimes you will experience blood-tinged vaginal discharge, also known as bloody show. Don't confuse this with losing your mucous plug. Your mucous plug is a big blob of mucus that forms in your cervix at the beginning of your pregnancy and comes out through your vagina, sometimes up to two weeks prior to going into labor. It serves as a barrier to prevent bacteria and infection from getting into your uterus. Not all women notice when this happens, and it's not the most reliable signal that it's time. There's also no need to collect your mucus plug to show your practitioner, you can flush it down the toilet. In all honesty, the mucous plug is really not a big deal, although some moms tend to make it out to be.

During this early phase, it is a great idea to take some walks with intermittent resting/napping as much as possible. You don't want to overdo it because your body is getting ready to switch into overdrive and you'll need all the energy you can muster soon enough. A warm shower or bath is a good way to help your body and muscles relax. Meditation and light stretching might also help. It's also very important to stay hydrated during this time and to eat small snacks to keep up those energy levels.

Water Breaking

One of the first signs that you're going on your way to having your baby is your water breaking; the amniotic membrane ruptures which allows the amniotic fluid to escape, known as spontaneous rupture of membranes (SROM). This can be a slow little trickle making you wonder about your bladder control, or it can be a gush (and you just changed the sheets!). To check if it's amniotic fluid spilling out of you, and not pee, give it a sniff. Amniotic fluid has a sweetish smell, whereas urine smells like ammonia, and well, pee. Most women will start having contractions if they aren't happening already. If they are, they may start to ramp up. Please note that not all women will have contractions on their own, water breaking or not. So, if you feel "leaking" or "wet", be sure to contact your healthcare provider. Use a pad or towel to contain the flow, don't use a tampon, and don't have sex.

Contact your practitioner immediately once the flow starts, and/or follow your labor and delivery protocol as discussed. When you get to the hospital, a sample of the fluid will likely be taken by inserting a cotton swab inside the vagina, having you cough a couple of times (making more fluid come out), and transferring the sample to a test tube. This will be sent to the lab to confirm whether it's amniotic fluid.

Sometimes the amniotic can be greenish-brown instead of clear. This could be due to meconium, the baby's very first "poop". Meconium is usually seen after birth but can be passed in-utero for various reasons. It's not necessarily a bad sign, but notify your practitioner of the color.

Your OB will likely want to induce contractions if they haven't already started. It used to be we would wait 24 hours for labor to naturally start, but studies have shown that if labor doesn't start within 4 hours of SROM, then it likely will not start on its own. Also, when your membranes are ruptured, there is a greater chance of getting an infection in utero. This would have you end up with a whole other set of problems. All practitioners have a different avenue of thought here, so again I would go with your provider's recommendation.

Don't be alarmed if your water doesn't break. Not every woman experiences it. Your practitioner will assist with breaking your water (AROM, or Artificial Rupture of Membranes), or augment your labor (help labor to continue progressing) when and if necessary.

Contractions

Contractions usually last 30 to 45 seconds and gradually increase in intensity and frequency up to five minutes apart. Remember, this phase can actually start to progress over several weeks prior to your due date when you don't even notice contractions happening. Starting off, contractions feel like menstrual cramps.

Not all women have textbook regular contractions. If your contractions vary in length and frequency, but they're long, (50 – 60) seconds, strong, and/or consistently 4 - 5 minutes apart, it's a very good sign that this is the real deal and not Braxton

Hicks contractions. When in doubt, assume it's the real thing and contact your practitioner. Don't worry about bothering your practitioner or think you might be wasting their time. Experienced practitioners can usually tell by your voice what phase of labor you're in. Head to the hospital after speaking to your provider if they feel you should go, or if your labor is so intense that you are not smiling anymore. Worst case scenario, we check you out and send you home if you're not in labor.

For some women, the first contractions pass unnoticed and painlessly, so that by the time they do feel the contractions, they're strong and frequent.

Other Signs and Symptoms of Labor:

- Backache
- Pressure in your lower abdomen
- Diarrhea
- Nausea/Vomiting

Stage One, Phase 2: Active Labor

Active labor is when the cervix dilates up to 7 – 8 cm. Contractions last a little bit longer, approximately 40 - 60 seconds, and are usually closer together, about 3 - 4 minutes apart. This is the time when your sweet smile switches to a blank look directed at your partner. Some women don't say a word, and some are very vocal at this point. There is no wrong way to express yourself in labor, you have every excuse to cuss and yell profanities if that's what you need to do. Your contractions will become more painful from here on out. You might also be experiencing excruciating back pain. If you need pain relief, don't be ashamed to ask for an epidural, it's there to help you make this experience as smooth as possible. Natural interventions that relieve back pain include ice packs, getting into the shower with warm water directed at the painful spot, using a birthing tub (if available), and counter pressure. Counter pressure is performed by applying significant pressure to the area of discomfort, whether it be the lower back or against the pelvic bones.

Planned a hospital or birth center birth? You should be on your way at the start of the active labor phase if you weren't already on the way at the end of your early phase.

Rocking back and forth with legs and hips open, and walking around can help alleviate some of the discomforts of the contractions and back pain. Leaning over a higher surface resting on pillows, sitting on a labor ball, kneeling, assisted squatting, lying on your side, or sitting in a tub can all possibly relieve some of the pressure off your pelvis while still keeping you as comfortable as possible. Some women like counterpressure either against their hips or on an area of their lower back. You can ask your support person to help aid with that.

Personally, I like to help my laboring mom focus on what is happening inside. Close your eyes, and visualize a round circle that is similar to when you blow up a balloon. As you blow, that circle (your cervix) opens and opens and opens a little bit at a time. If you can close your eyes and visualize as you blow gently, you're blowing up that balloon to complete dilation (10 cm) to allow baby to have an exit route.

Other Signs and Symptoms:

- Leg pain and discomfort (including the butt)
- Increasing bloody show
- Fatigue
- Water breaking (if it hasn't already happened)

If you're starting to feel lightheaded, or tingly in your toes, you could be hyperventilating. Tell a nurse, your midwife, or your doula, so that they can help you get your breathing back under control, or have you breathe into a paper bag to get those oxygen and carbon dioxide levels back to normal. Practicing slow breathing techniques early on can help with focus. Rhythmic breathing is performed by filling the abdomen first by inhaling for a count of 4 and then exhaling for a count of 8.

At the Hospital or Birthing Center

Unless it's an emergency, admission can take a while. To make the admission process as simple as possible, preregistration is recommended.

When you get to the unit, a nurse will take you either to a labor delivery recovery room (LDR), or an assessment room, and will then ask you if and when your water broke, when your contractions started, and other questions of a similar nature. You or your partner will be required to sign routine informed consent forms.

After this, you will be given a hospital gown to change into, and your vitals will be checked, namely blood pressure, temperature, pulse, respirations, and in some cases a urine sample. As explained before, an amniotic fluid sample may also be taken if your water has broken. Most hospitals will start an IV (especially if you want an epidural or if it's hospital policy), draw labs, and examine any bloody show or SROM. There are some moms that for whatever reason do not wish to have an IV. They will refuse unless they absolutely need it. That is fine and you are welcome to sign an AMA (Against Medical Advice) form. I do understand that a lot of women are low risk. But I have also seen women bleed out awfully fast during delivery or shortly after having a baby. An emergency in this situation can get ugly fast. The last thing you want is for us to struggle with getting an IV in during an emergency and your veins are nowhere to be seen due to severe blood loss. I do not want to alarm you, but instead, my intent here is to be sure you are informed.

To measure mom's contractions, a pressure-sensitive gauge called a TOCO (Tocodynamometer) is used. It is not a true reading of how strong the contractions are but instead can tell us *when* the contractions are and how the FHR (fetal heart rate) reacts to them.

The IUPC (intrauterine pressure catheter) is necessary to assess women who are being induced with Pitocin to determine whether the contractions are strong enough and close enough to determine the adequacy of labor. The IUPC is inserted along the inner wall of the uterus via SVE (sterile vaginal exam). Naturally, the uterine membrane of the mother must be ruptured to do this.

To monitor the baby's heart, practitioners can externally measure the baby's heart rate using an electronic fetal monitor (EFM). This is connected to the same monitor as the TOCO. Continued monitoring is mandatory when labor is induced or when the mother has received an epidural. As well, for women who are more at risk for complications, such as mothers with high blood pressure or diabetes, EFM is helpful as it can provide consistent information on how the baby is doing throughout labor in spite of said complication.

Intermittent monitoring (20 minutes out of every hour) with EFM is only recommended for low-risk births.

During the more intense pushing phase, the baby's heart rate will need to be continually monitored as well. Please know that we don't have the monitors on you to torture you further in labor and delivery. Not only is it our job to make sure you and your baby stay healthy during this arduous process, but many healthcare rules and regulations govern us, and we must chart everything we do. We can't chart it if we can't prove it, thus all the monitoring.

In cases where there is a concern for fetal distress, or that the practitioner is unable to monitor the baby for any reason, an electrode will be attached to the baby's head via SVE to assess their heart rate. These interventions do not "hurt" more than just the vaginal exam part of it.

Some hospitals have telemetry monitoring, where the EFM and TOCO are plugged into a portable machine that can transmit the baby's heartbeat and the mom's UCs (uterine contractions) to the monitor which is always being watched at the nurse's station, and still allows you to move around, walk the halls, etc.

Labor and delivery are like a beautiful dance. There are so many ways to ebb and flow. Every few hours your practitioner, midwife, or nurse will do an SVE to see how dilated your cervix is and the position of the baby. They'll also be timing your contractions and putting all the "dance moves" together. If labor isn't progressing, one way to "augment" your labor without the use of medications is through AROM. If induction is necessary, they'll then slowly administer oxytocin (Pitocin) to get those contractions going and your cervix dilating.

Stage One, Phase 3: Transitional Labor

Transition in labor is considered the most intense part of labor and gets you to a full 10 cm dilated. Contractions are now usually lasting 60 - 90 seconds and occur about every 2 - 3 minutes. This can take 15 minutes to an hour, but in some cases can go up to 3 - 5 hours. By now it probably feels like you've been in labor for eternity. There is much more pressure on your lower back, and perineum, along with rectal pressure, as your baby is moving down for delivery. You may or may not feel the urge to push, and it can feel like needing to go Number Two (or as some patients have said "I feel like I need to take the biggest poop of my life!").

Transition is physically and mentally demanding and exhausting, so hang in there. You've got this! If you're not completely dilated, you need to resist the urge to push. Pushing before your cervix is completely dilated can swell your cervix, thus prolonging the labor process. "Relax" is probably the last thing you want to hear now, and will likely earn the offender a punch, but try to get what rest you can in between contractions. Touches that might have been comforting a moment ago, like a soothing massage from your significant other, may feel like torture now. Cries of "don't touch me!" are common, express your needs to your birth team.

Nausea and/or vomiting, time distortion, hot or cold flashes (or both in turn), uncontrollable shaking, loss of modesty, cramping legs, drowsiness, intense exhaustion, and increasing irritability are all normal and part of the process. An epidural will and can bring relief should you need it.

Most importantly, remember why you're here! A beautiful baby is waiting for you on the other side of this ordeal!

Stage 2: Delivering the Baby

Congratulations Mama!

After all that hard work you'll probably be anxious to finally hold your little baby in your arms. The quicker practitioners can get the baby to mama, the better long-term outcomes for their sleeping, feeding, and overall well-being. The practitioner will get the baby's breathing and crying going and get them to you as soon as possible. That first skin-to-skin contact is magical, unforgettable, and essential. Your baby will eventually instinctively start sniffing out your breast to latch on and suckle.

While your baby is in your arms, the umbilical cord will be clamped and cut. If you have a cord blood kit, this is when and where the blood will be collected.

The nursery nurse or your delivery nurse will take the baby's first vitals while he/she is on your abdomen. Your baby will be evaluated and given an Apgar score. The Apgar score is a score total between 0 - 10 based on five different observations that are assessed, namely breathing, heart rate, muscle tone, reflex/grimace, and skin color, which are each given a score of 0 - 2. A perfect score would be 2 for each observation for a total of 10. This helps with the immediate care of the newborn but isn't indicative of the future well-being of your baby.

After your baby has nursed for the first time, or at least you have had some bonding time, your baby's first assessment will be done which includes more vitals, measurements including weight, as well as footprints. Identification bracelets will be attached to you, your partner, and the baby's ankle, and an antibiotic eye ointment will be given to prevent infection, as well as the Vitamin K injection. They will weigh your baby, then wrap them up nice and snug in a blanket to be returned to you. Or, they may just place the baby back skin to skin on your chest and cover it with baby blankets. Depending on the hospital, other pediatric examinations might occur now, or the following day if baby is healthy. Some hospitals still might have a nursery that all the babies go to in the morning for pediatrician assessments, otherwise, the pediatrician will make rounds to each patient's room to see and assess the sweet little babes. At this time, you can ask any questions you might have regarding your baby.

Once the baby's temperature is stable, you and your partner may be able to help to give your baby their first bath. Our birthing center has switched to giving the baby a bath after 24 hours, prior to discharge. Some parents opt to not have a baby bath at all as it removes any antimicrobial proteins that are beneficial for baby. This is something you can research on your own prior to delivery so that you can let the nursing staff know your wishes.

Stage 3: Delivering the Placenta

There are still a few small details to attend to before you're completely done. Any time after your baby's birth, your placenta will be expelled through mild contractions. This can last anywhere from 5 - 30 minutes. Your practitioner will help with this by applying pressure to your uterus, gently pulling the placenta out via the cord, and instructing you to push when necessary.

Afterward, the practitioner will examine the placenta to make sure it's intact, as well as manually examine the uterus for any bits left behind. It's incredibly important for the entirety of the placenta to be expelled, as anything left behind can cause continuous heavy bleeding or infection and other complications. If necessary, Pitocin will be administered to help deliver the entirety of the placenta. In some hospitals, it's part of their policy to always administer oxytocin to ensure that the entire placenta is expelled and bleeding is under control.

Did You Need Induction?

As I mentioned above, sometimes techniques need to be used or medication has to be administered to help things along. Medically induced labor is only done at a hospital or birthing center, while home birth is limited to natural techniques. Non-medication techniques used by healthcare professionals include:

- amniotomy, where a small hole is made in the amniotic sac to trigger your water breaking
- membrane stripping, where the practitioner gently separates the amniotic sac from the walls of the uterus to stimulate the release of prostaglandins
- Cervical Ripening Balloon induction, where a cervical ripening balloon is inserted into the cervix, and the inner and outer part is inflated like a balloon with a saline solution to trigger the release of prostaglandins

The type of medicinal induction depends on whether the cervix is ripe or not. Medications that are commonly used to induce labor are prostaglandins (misoprostol and dinoprostone), which "ripen" the cervix. Another medication, Pitocin (oxytocin), is also known as the parenting hormone. Oxytocin isn't just responsible for helping form that bond between you and your little one, another function is to contract the uterus to help push the baby, and later the placenta, out.

A ripe cervix is a cervix that has softened, started effacing, and started to dilate. If your cervix isn't ripe, and labor needs to be induced, the first step is administering prostaglandins. You will then be continuously monitored to see how things progress. If the cervix ripens and contractions begin, great! Hopefully, things start proceeding as normal from here. If your cervix ripens but contractions don't start, the next step is IV administration of Pitocin. If the cervix doesn't ripen with the first administration of prostaglandins, a second administration will follow. Your baby will be closely monitored throughout to make sure they remain healthy. If the prostaglandins fail to work, or Pitocin fails to trigger contractions, the practitioner will reevaluate and depending on the situation may opt for C-section.

For home births, possible techniques that can induce labor are:

- exercise
- sex
- nipple stimulation
- acupressure (just make sure you know what you're doing)
- eating dates (old wives' tale)
- spicy food (old wives' tale)

Please note, that although castor oil has long been believed to induce labor, there is very little medical evidence, and the side effects of drinking castor oil, nausea, vomiting, severe diarrhea, and dehydration, are not only uncomfortable but are also unnecessary risks at this point of the pregnancy. Never mind the mess for the nurses caring for you.

The most common reason for induction is if the baby is overdue, but induction can also be scheduled ahead of time for medical reasons listed below. When you've gone into labor by yourself but your contractions spaced out or labor just stopped, this is when your practitioner would "augment" your labor with Pitocin. Reasons for scheduling labor induction include:

- to ensure that you're at the hospital or birthing center once labor starts because you live far away
- the mother is diabetic
- the mother has high blood pressure
- the mother or the baby has other health complications that make it necessary
- the baby is growing too slowly

Other situations where labor is induced or augmented:

- the mother's water broke and there are no contractions within the next 24 hours
- contractions are irregular, not strong enough, not frequent enough
- if any part of the labor process is starting to take too long according to the practitioner
- oligohydramnios (not enough fluid)
- polyhydramnios (too much fluid)
- infection in the uterus
- premature rupture of membranes

Breastfeeding After Induction or Epidural

"I was told that the baby wouldn't be able to nurse if I have an epidural or pain medicine". First of all, that's not true. There are just as many babies born from unmedicated deliveries who have trouble nursing as there are babies born from medicated or induced delivery. Lactation and nursing are completely independent of how your baby was born. So, in a nutshell, do what is right for you and your family. Trust the process.

Of course, there are some women who simply can't breastfeed, whether because they don't produce enough milk, had to have a mastectomy, or some other factor. I have gone more into breastfeeding in *First-Time Parents: A Clear Guide and How-To for All Things Baby Birth - 1 Month.*

Cesarean Delivery

Whatever the reason you don't or can't opt for vaginal delivery, this doesn't make you a "weaker" or "worse" mother. Yes, there are pros to vaginal delivery, but there are also pros to C-sections. C-sections have saved thousands upon thousands of mothers and babies over the centuries, and ought to be respected just as much as vaginal delivery.

Why C-section?

There are many reasons why you or your practitioner decide on a C-section ahead of time and including:

- breech presentation or transverse position (if baby is not vertex, or "head down" or a part of the baby that's not the head will emerge first with vaginal delivery) could possibly lead to fetal injury or even death during vaginal birth

- if the mother is expecting multiple babies (some practitioners will attempt vaginal delivery of twins if they are both vertex)
- pre-eclampsia or eclampsia
- if the baby is too large to be delivered vaginally
- abnormal fetal heart rate
- obstruction
- previous C-section
- previous surgeries and or injuries of the abdominal area, pelvic area, and/or lower back (such as a pelvic fracture)
- placenta previa (where the placenta is too low in the uterus and blocks the cervix)
- preferring C-section over vaginal delivery
- some medical conditions, where pushing is not recommended

Sometimes, despite your best planning for a vaginal birth, you'll have to go for an unplanned C-section. This can happen due to:

- labor not progressing or taking too long to be considered safe
- if the baby at any point goes into fetal distress
- umbilical cord compression, where the cord wraps around the baby's neck or is pinched between the pelvis and the baby, causing suffocation
- umbilical cord prolapse, where the cord emerges before the baby

- placental abruption, where the placenta separates from the uterine wall before the baby's born
- failure to medically induce labor
- any situation where the practitioner deems it to be the best course for a healthy mama ~ healthy baby outcome

The Procedure

Unlike vaginal delivery, whether natural, induced, or under epidural, there's no pushing involved here. In fact, someone else will be doing the hard work for once. This surgical procedure usually only requires regional anesthesia, either through a spinal block (the anesthetic is injected into the subarachnoid space within the spine) or an epidural, numbing the lower half of the body. If a patient has been in labor and already has an epidural that has been working well, the anesthesiologist can usually use that same epidural to give an extra dose for complete numbing for surgery. In some cases, usually emergencies, C-section is performed under general anesthesia. With an epidural, you may still feel some tugging sensations as the surgery takes place, but there shouldn't be any pain.

Here is the step-by-step process:

- To start off, you'll be prepped for surgery, and an IV line will be attached to you for any necessary hydration, medication, or antibiotics.

- The anesthesia will now be given. If it's general anesthesia, you will be unconscious for the remainder of the procedure.
- Your abdomen will be wiped with an antiseptic solution to prevent infection once they start the incision, and a catheter will be inserted into your bladder (to keep it empty as you won't be feeling anything downstairs, making it harder to control things).
- Sterile drapes will be placed around your abdomen.
- A drape will be placed between you and your abdomen so that you won't see your own body being cut open. This is to keep the mother as calm and stress-free as possible in cases of regional anesthesia.
- If you have your partner or anyone else there to support you, they will scrub up (sanitize their hands and arms and wear sterile garbs, including a face mask) and be able to sit by you.
- Once the anesthetic has taken effect and is confirmed by the doctor, they will make an incision (usually a neat, horizontal one) just above the pubic hairline.
- The area of the incision is opened, and another incision is made in the uterus (also usually a horizontal one). The amniotic sac will be opened if it wasn't already ruptured, and the fluid will be suctioned out.
- The baby is then gently lifted out, while a nurse presses on the uterus. You can ask to see your baby if the drape

is blocking your view. Most drapes now have a "window" that can be used to show you the baby through.

- Any mucus will be suctioned from the baby's nose and mouth, their breathing will be stimulated, and you will hear their first cry. The cord will now also be clamped and cut.
- Baby is brought to the warmer for continued drying and assessment. Depending on the hospital, they might conduct the newborn examination before handing them to you.
- Once your baby is handed to you can have your skin-to-skin bonding like with vaginal delivery, the doctor will remove the placenta, do a routine check of your reproductive organs, and stitch you up. The uterus will be stitched with absorbable stitches, whilst your abdomen may be stitched, stapled, or glued shut.
- You will eventually feel the pain once the anesthesia wears off, you did undergo surgery after all. It may be difficult for you to move around because of the pain as well. Doctors will prescribe you safe pain medication. You will likely be staying in the hospital for two to four days for you to recover somewhat, and to monitor you and your baby.

Recovery

It can take four to six weeks for your body to recover from a C-section, while it takes only a few hours to a couple of days to recover from vaginal birth (if all went normally). This is one of the unfortunate downsides to having a C-section.

For the first day, you will need assistance getting into and out of bed. While you recover, you also shouldn't carry or pick up anything heavy. For once, exercise is a no-no. Any strenuous activity, including cleaning, cooking, and yes, sex, should be avoided. If you live in a house or apartment with stairs, see if you can convert any of the downstairs rooms into a temporary bedroom, if your bedroom isn't already on the ground floor. If you're a single parent, have a family member or close friend help you through this recovery period.

You will be in some pain, for which your doctor will prescribe pain medication that is safe to use alongside breastfeeding (if you are breastfeeding). Over-the-counter medications can also help, like good old Tylenol and ibuprofen. This is not a time for you to "be strong" and refuse pain medications if they are needed. To heal, you need to move so that you have good circulation which in turn will bring oxygen to your tissues, which helps with a quicker healing process. If you are in pain, you won't get up and move, so this process of healing will take much longer. There is no shame in taking pain medication if it's needed. Slowly but surely, you will wean off of it and feel normal again without it.

You'll also use sanitary pads (not tampons), as your uterus will be shedding, creating a vaginal discharge called lochia. The initial discharge will be red, and will gradually turn a yellow color. If you notice any abnormal coloration or bad smells, immediately contact your practitioner. Note: post deliver bleeding from a C-section will be much less than a vaginal delivery. It will be more like spotting.

Home Birth

Home birth, as the name says, means giving birth via vaginal delivery in the comfort and privacy of your own home. Home births are usually assisted by a qualified midwife and in some cases a family medicine doctor.

The idea of being surrounded by family and loved ones, no hospital bills, and welcoming your little one straight into their home is a wonderful one and is usually the reason why women want home births. Not everyone can safely deliver at home, however. It should only be considered by women who are perfectly healthy and at low risk.

If you're expecting more than one baby (twins, triplets), have any chronic condition like high blood pressure or diabetes, had a C-section in the past, or your baby is in the wrong position, or has any health problems, you should deliver at a hospital or birthing center.

Keep in mind, however, that there are no IVs, no epidurals, and no other medical interventions at home. It's just you, your midwife, your doula (if you have one), and whoever else is invited to the birthday party.

The pros of home birth are:

- freedom of movement and being able to do what you want
- privacy
- no hospital bills
- increased bonding with your baby
- more family and friends can be involved
- smaller risk of infections to the mother
- comfortable and familiar environment
- can do water birth

Set up a birth plan for your home birth, including whom you want to be there, where you want to give birth, what you want for comfort and to be able to relax, and how you'll manage pain. Your midwife most likely (hopefully) has done many home births and will be able to give you the process of how it will all go. It's also important to have contingency plans in place, such as access and transportation to a hospital in case of an emergency. Have a hospital bag packed just in case.

You should get to the hospital immediately when:

- labor is taking too long
- the baby is in the wrong position
- your blood pressure is high
- you have a fever

- there is excessive bleeding
- you need pain relief
- the baby is in distress

I think homebirth can be a beautiful thing. I have several friends that have had one. But it is hard for someone who has been in obstetrics for many years, in a hospital setting, to fully recommend this way of delivery. Yes, I have seen many beautiful, uncomplicated births over the years, but I have also seen births that became complicated over the labor and/or delivery process. Not to mention, the many "failed home births" and sometimes tragedies that end up at the hospital. I don't say this to scare you, but to be completely transparent. Personally, I would never take that chance. If you absolutely despise hospitals, then just go have your baby there and leave AMA early, but after you are recovered and there are no signs of a problem. I would rather see you surrounded by emergency personnel and equipment in the event of an emergency than not. Ultimately, you need to make the right decision for yourself and your family.

Water Birth

This involves going through labor and delivering the baby in a tub of water. The water takes some of the pressure off the mother and can alleviate some of the pain. Most water births take place at home. Not many hospitals or birthing centers give the option, due to hygiene and safety concerns.

Water births carry all the risks of home births, along with a few of their own unique risks:

- Drowning: There's water, so the baby and/or you can drown due to complications or a freak accident.
- Increased risk of infection: Water is a natural breeding ground for bacteria, and add to that a combination of your own bodily fluids and quite possibly feces, this creates a less than hygienic environment that can make your baby sick.
- Meconium aspiration: This happens when the baby inhales some amniotic fluid containing meconium. This naturally causes breathing issues after birth and can cause infections like pneumonia.
- Umbilical cord tear: Babies are naturally buoyant, and so the baby will shoot up to the surface once they've been pushed out of the cervix. The force is sometimes enough to cause the cord to tear, which will lead to life-threatening bleeding. The cord should be clamped as soon as possible, and the baby will likely have anemia afterward.

We did water births at the first hospital I worked at as a young nurse. They were beautiful and calming deliveries. The biggest problem I saw was getting mom and baby out of the water to the bed. And it was only a messy problem.

At the hospital I am at currently, we do have labor tubs for use during labor, but moms are instructed to get to the bed for delivery. Sometimes they don't make it. Oops! I will say, labor tubs are amazing for comfort during labor. My favorite doula and I have great success having quick natural labors using the labor tub. Usually, your nurse will allow you to use the tub when you get to 5 cm or so. Too much earlier and it may get you to relax too much that your labor will stall. Of course, if you are on Pitocin then we can make sure your contractions continue. However, you cannot be on Pitocin without being continuously monitored, so hopefully, you are at a facility that was telemetry.

Vaginal Delivery vs. Cesarean Delivery

As I've mentioned, there are reasons for both methods, and both methods are valid. Here I will provide a brief summary of the pros and cons for ease of comparison. At-risk mothers will nearly always be recommended for cesarean delivery, however, so keep that in mind.

	Vaginal	**Cesarean**
Recovering from pain after birth	Short recovery	Long recovery (6 - 8 weeks)
Hospital Stay	Short stay (24 - 48 hours)	Long stay (2 - 4 days)
Surgical risks	None	Present
Delivery time	Long	Short
Risk of pelvic injuries and vaginal tears	Present	None
Risk to baby getting injured	Higher	Lower
Timing of delivery	Unpredictable	Basically, always on time
Risk of urinary incontinence	Higher	Lower
Intensity of labor	High	None
Risk of blood clots	Lower	Higher
Control over the safety of the process	Lower	Higher
Risk of respiratory problems in the baby	Lower	Higher

How Does Your Baby Look?

You won't be able to see if your baby has your eyes or if they're biological fathers just yet, but there are a few other things you can ooh and aah over now that you have unrestricted viewing access to your little angel.

- **Should their head look like that?** If you're referring to any weird shapes your baby's head may have after vaginal delivery, yes, that's normal. They had to be squeezed through a small space, and their flexible skull enabled them to do so, which might give it a pointed, cone-like shape. The skull will settle into its normal shape over the next two weeks. Babies delivered via C-section had no squeezing to do, so their heads are the expected round shape, unless you had to push for 4 hours prior to having a cesarean section.
- **Bald or billowing locks?** Depending on genetic factors, your baby may be born with only a few wisps of downy hair, or a thick bush of curls. Their newborn hair will eventually make way for their baby hair, but keep that little head warm with a cute hat anyway.
- **Fluffy or waxy coat:** Babies born earlier may still have their vernix and/or lanugo coating. These will be shed soon enough. Overdue babies are highly likely to have shed their coats already.

- **Skin color:** Your baby might be paler, or even more purple than you'd expect. This is because your baby's skin pigmentation hasn't settled in yet. Jaundice is also common, no need to worry. Most babies' jaundice clears up by itself, but if needed, they can soak under a special light that helps to break down bilirubin (the substances causing jaundice). Your baby may also be sporting a birthmark somewhere on their body, or even rashes that will quickly disappear.
- **Puffy eyes:** Other than being disturbed from a nice and relaxing 9-month holiday, your baby's eyes will be puffy from soaking in amniotic fluid. This too will pass.
- **Eye color:** Most babies are born with dark-brown eyes, or slate blue-gray eyes, that will eventually turn the color they inherited from you or their biological father as the pigmentation settles.

5

Expecting Multiples

Multiple pregnancy is when a mother is expecting more than one baby. Usually, this refers to twins and triplets, and also includes quadruplets, quintuplets, and even more! Expecting multiples is a unique experience and very special, but can lead to possible complications due to various factors. Before you get the torch and pitchfork, this doesn't mean that the babies themselves are the complications unless you count the financial complication of budgeting for one baby and getting a surprise at your first ultrasound. It's recommended to deliver multiples via C-section to ensure the safest delivery for all the babies and mama. Some practitioners will deliver twins if both present vertex at the time of delivery. Or, if at least the first is head down, they can use an ultrasound to turn the 2nd baby after the first is delivered. Of course, this is done in the C-section room in case of emergency.

All multiples are either because a fertilized egg split before implanting, or when more than one egg cell was released and fertilized. There are a number of reasons why this will happen, namely:

- family history of multiples and/or being a twin or triplet
- fertility treatment that stimulates ovulation and the release of multiple egg cells
- older maternity age
- random chance

Types of Multiples

Identical (Monozygotic)

Most people have met identical twins or seen them on tv, and they often draw a lot of curiosity and fascination because of their physical similarities, similar personalities, and close relationships. As I explained above, some multiples are caused by a fertilized egg cell splitting. This is what leads to identical multiples. A single split will lead to identical twins, while two splits will lead to triplets, and so forth. Identical multiples are always the same sex and are always similar in appearance. The reason for this is that all identical multiples share the same genome, in other words, they are genetically practically identical.

Fraternal (Dizygotic)

When more than one egg cell is available and fertilized by different sperm, fraternal twins, triplets, and more are the result. These babies are not identical and can be of different sexes. Essentially, they differ genetically as much as siblings who are born in different years. IVF has a high chance of resulting in fraternal multiples as a number of fertilized eggs are transferred to the uterus which is the reason for more multiple pregnancies in recent years.

Types of Separation

The type of multiples, and in the case of identical multiples, the timing when the fertilized egg cell split, will determine if individual placentas and/or amniotic sacs will develop for each multiple. For example, fraternal twins always develop their own separate placenta and amniotic sac, whereas a fertilized egg cell that divides after one week will have one placenta, but individual amniotic sacs.

Monochorionic-Diamniotic

This translates directly to one shared placenta and two amniotic sacs. Most identical twins (70%) present as monochorionic-diamniotic, with each baby developing in their own amniotic sac, but sharing the placenta with their sibling. It's almost always identical twins when this type of separation is present. Due to sharing a placenta, there's a chance for twin-to-twin transfusion.

Monochorionic-Monoamniotic

In other words, one shared placenta, and one shared amniotic sac. These are always identical multiples who share a single placenta and a single amniotic sack with their siblings. In this type of separation, there's an even greater chance of twin-to-twin transfusion, as well as oligohydramnios or polyhydramnios, and the risk of miscarriage is much larger.

Dichorionic-Diamniotic

Literally, two placentas and two amniotic sacs. This is the most viable form of separation, where each baby develops with its own placenta and its own amniotic sac. Most multiples separated this way are fraternal, but identical multiples can also present with dichorionic-diamniotic separation. For this reason, the risks are lower compared to other multiples, but still higher than expecting a single baby.

Signs and Symptoms

Aside from seeing more than one baby with your first ultrasound, and hearing more than one heartbeat during the Doppler scan, there are other early signs that could indicate that you're expecting multiples.

- More severe nausea and vomiting. Sadly, yes, double babies mean double the trouble for some symptoms.
- Faster weight gain during pregnancy. You are carrying more than one baby after all, and both are growing at relatively the same rate.

- Higher hCG levels. More hCG will be produced with the bonus baby (or babies) on board.
- High amounts of alpha-fetoprotein (AFP). in your blood. AFP is normally measured to screen for the presence of Down syndrome and neural tube effects, but because AFP correlates with fetal serum, high levels of AFP are indicative of multiples.

Women expecting multiples usually also appear much larger during their pregnancy, as she very likely is. The more babies, the more space is taken up.

Complications:

Expecting just one baby can have many complications and difficulties, so adding another baby or two into the mix just increases the risks.

Preterm Labor and Birth

This is the most common complication when expecting multiples. Due to the combined weight of multiples, labor is likely to start earlier than standard pregnancies. The ideal timeframe for multiples is for the mother to go into labor at week 37. Babies from multiple pregnancies are therefore smaller than most babies from single pregnancies born full term and are thus at risk of low birth weight.

Preeclampsia

A woman's blood pressure is likely to increase during single pregnancy but in some cases, it can reach dangerous levels (over 140/90 mmHg). When expecting multiples, blood pressure rises even more, and therefore the risk of developing preeclampsia is much higher and is also likely to develop earlier during pregnancy. For more on the risks and dangers of preeclampsia, see chapter 6, *Complications*.

Gestational Diabetes

Even though the exact cause of gestational diabetes is unknown, it's theorized that the increased levels of certain hormones are contributing factors. With multiples, there are even higher levels of hormones, due to a larger placenta or even multiple placentas.

Placenta Abruption

When the placenta detaches from the uterus before delivery, it's a medical emergency as both the mother and the babies can die. Due to the increased weight and pressure of multiples, the risk of placental abruption is higher.

Fetal Growth Restriction (FGR)

As the name implies, babies don't grow at the expected or healthy rate. This leads to the possibility that babies are born preterm, have low birth weight and may have developmental abnormalities. In half of all multiple pregnancies, at least one of the babies has FGR due to having to share space and recourses.

Twin-to-Twin Transfusion Syndrome

This rare condition can affect monochorionic multiples. With twin-to-twin transfusion syndrome (TTTS), the veins and arteries providing blood and nutrients to the developing babies aren't evenly distributed. The one twin, the donor twin, transfers more blood than it receives, whilst the other twin, the recipient twin, receives more blood than they transfer.

For the donor twin, this can lead to malnutrition, low growth rate, decreased bladder size, and possibly organ failure. They're also more at risk of oligohydramnios due to less urination, cardiovascular problems, and death.

For the recipient twin, this can lead to other complications, such as overstimulating the heart and abnormal growth rate. Overstimulating the heart can lead to heart failure, which can end in the baby's death. Additionally, they are at risk of polyhydramnios.

A practitioner can pick up signs of TTTS through routine ultrasound and can conduct further tests to determine amniotic fluid volume, as well as each twin's heart function. If the diagnosis is confirmed, it's essential to continue monitoring the twins' heart function.

The Quintero staging system is used to assess the severity of TTTS.

- Stage 1 determines the presence of oligohydramnios and/or polyhydramnios.
- Stage 2 determines the size and visibility of the donor twin's bladder.
- Stage 3 assesses blood imbalance and heart function. In the case of heart failure, immediate intervention is necessary to save the baby.
- Stage 4 presents with fetal hydrops, a dangerous amount of fluid that gathers inside two or more parts of the baby (edema), putting additional stress on the heart and other organs
- Stage 5 is when at least one of the twins has passed away.

A relatively recent treatment method has been developed, called fetoscopic laser photocoagulation (FLP). Only a few medical centers in the U.S. can perform FLP however. Depending on the characteristics of each case of TTTS, either the relevant connections between the twins are ablated, or the placenta is functionally divided in two. Although the method isn't failsafe and can cause pain and discomfort to the mother, it's the best intervention for TTTS, particularly during Stage 2 and Stage 4.

The risks of FLP:

- Preterm birth
- PROM
- Bleeding
- Separation of the amniotic sac from the placenta
- Accidental damage to surrounding tissue
- Death of one or both of the babies

Twin-Anemia-Polycythemia Sequence

Twin-anemia-polycythemia sequence (TAPS) is a condition that also affects monochorionic twins. In this condition, the amniotic volume for both twins stays the same, but due to dysfunction in the blood exchange between them, one twin will become anemic (low amount of red blood cells), while the cotwin will become polycythemic (high amount of red blood cells). This can usually only be picked up by Doppler examination, which will pick up abnormalities in blood circulation. Spontaneous TAPS refers to the condition developing on its own, whilst it can develop in 16% of cases following FLP treatment of TTTS.

At present, the main treatment options are FLP, expectant management, preterm delivery, blood transfusions in-utero, and selective reduction.

The risks and long-term expectations are similar to that of TTTS.

Selective Fetal Growth Restriction

As the name implies, one of the babies' growth gets restricted, while the other develops normally. This is once again due to the unequal distribution of oxygen and nutrients between monochorionic twins, causing one twin to grow better than the other. This can only be picked up via ultrasound.

The growth-restricted twin can suffer severe growth and developmental deficiencies, as well as a high risk of death. It differs from TTTS in that amniotic volume remains unaffected.

There are three types of sFGR based on the direction of blood flow:

- Type 1: Forward flow of blood in the umbilical cord artery of the growth-restricted twin.
- Type 2: Either no blood flow or reversal of blood flow in the umbilical cord artery of the growth-restricted twin.
- Type 3: Unpredictable flow of blood in the umbilical cord of the growth-restricted twin.

Treatment of sFGR depends on the type.

With Type 1, the mother will be monitored weekly. If it progresses to Type 2 or Type 3, treatment will progress accordingly.

Type 2 and Type 3 are treated with selective cord occlusion. If sFGR has progressed to this stage, then the health and outcome of the unrestricted twin will be prioritized. For this reason, a small surgery will be done to stop blood flow to the growth-restricted twin. This is done with bipolar cord coagulation or radiofrequency ablation. This can lead to preterm labor.

Twin-Reversed-Arterial-Perfusion Syndrome

This rare condition also only affects monochorionic twins. With twin-reversed-arterial-perfusion syndrome (TRAP), only one twin's heart is functional and pumping to deliver blood to both. Sadly, the twin who does not have a functional heart (pump twin) will not survive delivery. The twin whose heart is functional also needs to do double the work and can put their heart under extreme stress and possibly failure. This is detectable by ultrasound.

To save the pump twin, bipolar cord coagulation or radiofrequency ablation are used to block blood flow to the acardiac twin.

Conjoined Twins

This refers to twins who are physically connected to each other. This is likely due to the partial splitting of the embryo. Conjoined twins may share organs as well. Most conjoined twins are stillborn or have a low life expectancy after birth.

Depending on how the twins are conjoined, they can be surgically separated. In some cases, one twin has to be surgically removed to ensure the survival of the other.

The twins are usually connected at the following sites:

- Chest
- Abdomen
- The base of the spine
- Along the length of the spine
- Pelvis
- Upper body
- Head
- Head and chest

6

Complications

No one likes complications. We want to keep pregnancy and delivery as complication-free as possible. Most can be prevented by being healthy and responsible. It's up to you how much you want to read up on everything that can potentially go wrong, and it's recommended to do this before you're pregnant, as any unnecessary worry and stress are to be avoided. It's good to have a general idea of what to look out for, but it's also important not to become paranoid and look for problems where there are none. If you're ever worried or in doubt, contact your practitioner.

Complications During Pregnancy

Although I've already covered a few in previous chapters, I'll mention them here again to be succinct.

Cervical Incompetence

Also known as cervical insufficiency is a condition due to weak cervical tissue. This poses a risk for preterm birth and pregnancy loss.

The symptoms are:

- light vaginal bleeding
- changes in vaginal discharge
- lower back pain (that hasn't been there before)
- a feeling of pressure on the pelvis
- abdominal cramps

Factors that can increase your risk of getting cervical incompetence:

- previous trauma to the cervix, such as previous surgery or an unusual Pap smear
- ethnicity, women of African heritage are at greater risk
- genetic disorders that affect body tissue development

Prevention:

- healthy lifestyle
- frequent prenatal checkups
- managing weight gain during pregnancy

Fetal Growth Restriction (FGR)

Also called intrauterine growth restriction (IUGR). This condition is characterized by abnormal growth rates of the baby during pregnancy, so they have lower birth weights (weighing approximately 10% less than healthy babies of the same age). There are two kinds, symmetrical FGR (the baby's entire body and head are smaller), and unsymmetrical FGR (the baby's head is of healthy size, but the body is smaller).

This is caused by insufficient oxygen and nutrient supply to the baby via the placenta and/or umbilical cord. Practitioners pick it up through routine checkups and ultrasounds and will continue to monitor it throughout the pregnancy.

Factors that affect the pregnant mother can increase the risk of the baby developing FGR. These include:

- smoking and/or drinking during pregnancy
- infections such as toxoplasmosis and German measles
- certain medications (such as epilepsy medication)
- autoimmune conditions such as lupus
- other chronic conditions such as anemia
- high blood pressure
- carrying multiples

Other risks for the baby:

- low immunity
- abnormal blood counts
- respiratory problems
- neurological problems
- difficulty suckling/feeding
- difficulty managing body temperature

The only treatment is for the mother to eat healthily and manage her weight gain during pregnancy. The practitioner will determine whether induction or C-section will be necessary for the baby's delivery, and at what gestational age.

Gestational Diabetes:

It's in the name. This is a condition where a mother develops diabetes during pregnancy, and it usually goes away after the baby is born. Just as with Diabetes Type I and Type II, gestational diabetes is associated with high blood sugar levels and insulin problems.

The symptoms are hard to catch, with some women experiencing increased thirst and the need to pee more. The only way to truly know if you have it is by doing frequent blood glucose tests.

The exact cause of gestational diabetes is unknown, but there are known risk factors that can contribute to women developing it during pregnancy:

- obesity
- physical inactivity
- family history of diabetes
- unhealthy diet
- insulin resistance

Risks to the mother due to gestational diabetes:

- higher blood pressure and preeclampsia
- developing future diabetes

Risks to the baby due to gestational diabetes:

- preterm birth
- high birth weight (9 pounds and more)
- breathing difficulties
- hypoglycemia (low blood sugar)
- stillbirth
- diabetes later in life

Gestational diabetes is usually treated with lifestyle changes, such as a healthy diet and exercise. Medication, such as metformin tablets or insulin injections, is only taken when necessary.

Hyperemesis Gravidarum (HG)

In layman's terms, this is excessive and abnormal vomiting during pregnancy and needs hospital treatment. Only 0,5 - 2% of pregnant ever experience HG.

It's different from normal sickness as the vomiting is so severe, that it causes dehydration, impairment of everyday functioning, and low weight gain during pregnancy. It's also associated with low blood pressure and elevated pulse.

The likeliest cause of HG is abnormal levels of hCG during pregnancy.

Symptoms of HG:

- constant nausea
- very frequent vomiting
- loss of appetite and difficulty keeping anything down
- weight loss due to vomiting or lack of eating
- dehydration
- lightheadedness and dizziness

Risk factors for HG:

- family history of HG
- first pregnancy
- expecting multiples

HG is treated in the hospital by attaching you to an IV to keep you hydrated. Due to the risks posed by dehydration and weight loss caused by HG, medication will also be given, such as promethazine.

Infections

Group B Streptococcus

The most common infection to affect mothers and their babies is group B streptococcus bacterial infection (GBS). Most mothers carrying GBS don't transmit it to their babies, but a small number of incidences do occur where the baby gets infected during birth. In other rare situations, it can cause miscarriage, preterm birth, or stillbirth.

If you're found to be carrying GBS, you will need to be given antibiotics (usually penicillin unless you're allergic) via your IV during labor to prevent transmission to your baby. After delivery, your baby will be monitored for any signs and symptoms of infection. If a baby is infected, they're very likely to recover with medical treatment. In some cases, however, it can progress to more dangerous infections, such as meningitis.

Babies can either have early-onset GBS infection, within 24 hours after birth or late-onset GBS infection, weeks or months after birth.

Symptoms of GBS infection in your baby:

- difficulty breathing
- limp and unresponsive body
- high or low temperature
- fussy and crying a lot
- difficulty feeding and vomiting
- rapid or slow heart rate
- rapid or slow breathing
- changes in skin color

Urinary Tract Infections

Women are generally more vulnerable to developing UTIs due to having a shorter urethra compared to men. UTIs are caused by foreign bacteria entering the urethra, or an overgrowth of the naturally occurring bacteria in the body, in other words, a disturbance in the natural bacterial balance. Lactobacilli are "good" bacteria naturally occurring in the vagina, along with anaerobic bacteria. Bacterial overgrowth can be caused by not urinating frequently, changes in pH (often due to using incorrect hygiene products), being immune compromised, or natural predilection to UTIs.

Women are even more vulnerable when they're pregnant because the baby puts more pressure on the bladder and urethra, along with all the physical and hormonal changes in the body. Urine also becomes more concentrated during pregnancy, causing a more favorable environment for bacterial growth.

UTIs are risky if untreated, as they can lead to preterm birth, the development of more serious infections, and complications during delivery.

The following can prevent you from contracting a UTI:

- urinating frequently and going when you need to go
- avoid using douches, perfumed sprays, and soap in and around your vagina (rinsing with water is enough to keep it clean). A bubble bath and bath salts are also to be avoided as they can cause pH changes
- drink a lot of water and stay hydrated
- wear clean, cotton underwear

Symptoms to look out for:

- burning or painful sensation when urinating
- blood in the urine or cloudy urine
- fever
- nausea and vomiting
- lower back and pelvic pain
- frequent need to urinate

UTIs are to be treated with antibiotics that are safe to use during pregnancy, such as nitrofurantoin, and cephalosporins. Ampicillin used to be the drug of choice, but bacteria have become more resistant to it in recent years.

Bacterial Vaginosis

As the name implies, this is a bacterial infection of the vagina. As discussed under UTIs, there are normal, naturally occurring bacteria inside the vagina. When the ratio between the bacteria is disturbed, if the number of anaerobe bacteria increases, this can lead to bacterial vaginosis. This mild infection is easily treated, with few symptoms, but the most common symptom is foul-smelling vaginal discharge.

Bacterial vaginosis can cause the following complications during pregnancy:

- preterm birth
- low birth weight

- increased risk of developing sexually transmitted infections (STIs)
- increased risk of developing pelvic inflammatory disease (PID)
- increased risk of infection after surgery, including C-sections

Bacterial vaginosis can be prevented by many of the measures used to prevent UTIs, namely:

- avoid using douches, perfumed sprays, and soap in and around your vagina, bubble bath, and bath salts
- wear clean, cotton underwear
- use protection during sex, especially if you have multiple sexual partners

Prescription medication to treat bacterial vaginosis include:

- metronidazole
- tinidazole
- clindamycin

Cytomegalovirus

This is a common infection that is normally harmless. It's related to the viruses that cause chicken pox and cold sores, which means that it stays in the body for the rest of your life once you're first infected. If a woman is infected with the virus while pregnant, however, it can be transmitted to the baby, who doesn't have a developed immune system yet.

Not all babies who have cytomegalovirus have any symptoms after birth. A few babies may develop hearing problems, or even trouble with their sight, later on, despite showing no early signs.

Babies who are born sick from cytomegalovirus present with the following symptoms:

- low birth weight
- preterm birth
- jaundice
- enlarged dysfunctional liver (hence jaundice)
- enlarged spleen
- rash or purple splotches on the skin
- small head
- pneumonia
- seizures

Adults with a functioning immune system don't require any medical treatment and usually recover from the infection on their own, and only experience flu-like symptoms. Babies and individuals with a weak immune system, who become sick from cytomegalovirus, need to be treated or it can be fatal.

Cytomegalovirus is transmitted through bodily fluids, so to prevent contracting it the following measures can be followed:

- wash your hands with soap and water
- regularly wash things that may have been in contact with bodily fluids (toys, cutlery, underwear, etc.)

- avoid sharing food, drinks, and cutlery with others
- avoid close contact with people with flu-like symptoms

Hepatitis B Virus

The hepatitis B virus (HBV) causes serious liver infections. Although most adults can recover from HBV, chronic HBV (HBV lasting longer than 6 months) can lead to liver failure, liver cirrhosis, and/or liver cancer. In children, HBV can develop into a lifelong condition. A mother can transmit HBV to her baby during pregnancy. The greatest risk posed by HBV to the unborn baby is for them to die prematurely of liver failure or cirrhosis, or they may develop serious liver diseases later in life.

HBV can be prevented by receiving an HBV vaccine before traveling to at-risk countries. If you've visited a country with a high prevalence of HBV, or live in a country where it's prevalent, it's important to screen for HBV before becoming pregnant, and during pregnancy. There is no cure for HBV, but the symptoms can be treated. A newborn whose mother has HBV needs to receive the HBV vaccine as soon as possible, ensuring the greatest effectiveness.

Most symptoms of HBV start one to four months after becoming infected, although some people may experience no symptoms. Signs and symptoms to look out for:

- fever
- jaundice

- joint pain
- weakness and fatigue
- abdominal pain
- dark urine
- loss of appetite
- abdominal pain

It's paramount to seek medical care if you know you've been exposed to HBV.

Influenza / The Flu

Most people have had the flu at some point in their life, and it's not a fun experience. Having the flu while pregnant, however, can be deadly for the mother and the baby, as it impacts the immune system, heart, and lungs.

The greatest risks to the baby include:

- preterm birth
- low birth weight
- stillbirth

The greatest risks to the mother include:

- middle ear infection
- developing meningitis
- inflammation of the brain (encephalitis)
- Inflammation of the heart (endocarditis)
- developing septic shock

The last four are particularly dangerous and can be lethal.

It's vital for mothers to get the flu shot, and it's perfectly safe to take during pregnancy. The vaccine can prevent becoming infected with the influenza virus, or if the mother does become infected, leads to less serious symptoms.

The best treatment for the flu is to treat the symptoms, lots of bed rest, stay warm, and drink plenty of water. Antiviral treatment can lessen the recovery time but doesn't treat the infection immediately.

To avoid getting the flu, get vaccinated as well as:

- avoid the outdoors as much as possible during the winter
- avoid crowded locations and contact with sick people
- wash your hands frequently and avoid touching your face
- stay home when you feel sick

Yeast Infection

Yeast infections are normally caused by changes in the pH balance of the vagina. It's fairly common during pregnancy, as hormonal changes can cause pH changes downstairs. The most common symptoms are vaginal itching and a thick, cottage cheese-like discharge.

Preventative measures for yeast infections are the same as for preventing UTIs and bacterial vaginosis. Basically, avoid using douches, perfumed soaps and sprays, bubble baths, and bath salts, and wear clean, cotton underwear.

Antifungal treatments in the form of cream, ointment, or suppositories are safe to use during pregnancy. Medications available in these forms are miconazole, clotrimazole, and terconazole. Oral antifungal treatments, like fluconazole, are to be avoided.

Although not a very serious condition to the mother, yeast infections can be transmitted to the baby. They usually develop an infection in the mouth (oral thrush) or diaper area, but in serious cases can spread throughout the body, causing heart and lung problems. It can also cause preterm birth.

Toxoplasmosis

This is a relatively common infection that usually passes without any symptoms. If symptoms are experienced, they're flu-like.

Toxoplasmosis does however pose a risk during pregnancy, particularly if the infection is contracted during later pregnancy. If the infection is transferred to the baby, it can cause miscarriage, stillbirth, or birth defects.

The infection can be contracted from the ground, improperly cooked meat, and cat poop. Thus, pregnant women are advised to:

- wear gloves while gardening
- ensure that meat and fish are cooked properly, so no sushi or raw cooked steak while pregnant
- wash all knives, cutting boards, and other utensils that have been used to prepare raw meat or fish - don't use the same knife that's been used for meat or fish to cut up other things before washing either
- ask your partner to take over litter box duty in the meantime, otherwise ask a friend, family member, or neighbor to help out (if all else fails, wear gloves and wash your hands thoroughly afterward)
- screen your cat for toxoplasmosis, and if they test positive, have someone look after them until they're clean
- wash fruit and vegetables thoroughly
- only use pasteurized dairy
- make sure your water is filtered, clean, and safe to drink
- if you have children who love playing in sandboxes, ensure that they wash up afterward, and if it's your own sandbox, regularly replace the sand with sterile sand

If you've already had toxoplasmosis, you'll be naturally immune and won't pose any threat to your baby. It can't be transferred between people outside of the uterus either, and you can't catch it directly from petting a cat.

If you do become infected while pregnant, the doctor can prescribe spiramycin, or a combination of pyrimethamine and sulfadiazine.

Oligohydramnios

This is a condition where the amniotic fluid volume is too low in relation to the baby's gestational age. The correct volume is necessary to protect the baby in many ways. The amniotic fluid acts as a shock absorber, protects the baby from infection, prevents the umbilical cord from compressing, allows the baby to move around, regulates their temperature, and also helps to develop their digestive tract and respiratory system. The amount of amniotic fluid can be measured via ultrasound, which will be done during regularly scheduled consultations with the practitioner. After Week 24, the AFI will also be measured (see chapter 3, *What to Expect, The Good, The Bad, and Staying Healthy*, under *Checkups During the Second Trimester*).

Oligohydramnios is uncommon, and most cases occur in the final three months, or when the baby is overdue.

Signs and symptoms are:

- small uterus measurements
- the baby doesn't move often
- clear fluid leaks from the vagina
- not enough weight gain during pregnancy

Possible causes:

- diabetes
- hypertension and preeclampsia
- genetic abnormalities

- placental problems
- PROM
- dehydration
- twin-to-twin transfusion syndrome
- pregnancy lasting two weeks past the due date

If oligohydramnios happens early in pregnancy, it can sometimes cause dangerous complications to the baby, namely:

- growth deformities
- miscarriage
- stillbirth
- preterm birth
- FGR
- umbilical cord compression
- underdeveloped respiratory and digestive systems
- increased risk of infection if the water breaks early

If the mother is diagnosed with oligohydramnios, the approach will depend on how far the pregnancy has progressed and if other complications are present. If the pregnancy is close to full-term (anywhere from week 37), the practitioner may recommend inducing labor if it's safe to do so. Otherwise, the practitioner will continue to monitor the mother and pregnancy closely to intervene when necessary. During labor, an amnioinfusion may be done, which is when fluid is added to the uterus during labor to prevent umbilical cord collapse and other complications. The fluid is transferred via catheter, and usually consists of saline or lactated Ringer's solution. Oligohydramnios does increase the possibility for delivery via C-section, however.

Polyhydramnios

The opposite of oligohydramnios, polyhydramnios is a condition where there is too much amniotic fluid present. It's not as serious as oligohydramnios, but extra monitoring will be necessary just in case.

Most cases of polyhydramnios lead to healthy births, but there is a risk of the following:

- preterm birth
- stretching of the uterus, which can cause severe bleeding after birth
- water breaking early
- problems with umbilical cord positioning and increased risk of umbilical cord prolapse
- possible health problems for the baby

There usually aren't noticeable symptoms for polyhydramnios, but some women may experience:

- swollen ankles and feet
- feeling out of breath
- constipation
- heartburn

Possible causes:

- diabetes and gestational diabetes
- expecting multiples
- infection during pregnancy
- the baby inherits a genetic condition

The only treatments for polyhydramnios are to treat the underlying causes and to possibly adjust the mother's birth plan if necessary. The mother should ensure to get enough rest and report any new symptoms as soon as possible. Labor can usually progress normally, and if necessary, labor will be induced, or C-section will be performed. Babies will be examined for any possible health problems after birth.

Preterm Labor

Preterm labor is defined as labor starting before week 37 of pregnancy. Not all cases of preterm labor lead to preterm birth if handled correctly. Numerous factors can cause preterm labor, such as:

- expecting multiples
- a shortened cervix
- other complications of pregnancy
- history of preterm labor
- stress and major life events
- age (very young and first-time mothers, as well as older mothers, are more at risk)

- past gynecological problems
- previous surgery in the pelvic region
- chronic conditions like high blood pressure and diabetes
- smoking during pregnancy
- vaginal bleeding
- infections of the uterus or lower genital tract

The biggest risk of preterm labor, is preterm birth, as the baby will not be fully developed and ready, which can cause an entirely different set of compilations for the baby.

Placenta Problems:

There are five placental problems that can lead to complications during pregnancy. These are:

Placental insufficiency:

When the placenta isn't correctly attached to the uterus, this will cause insufficient transfer of oxygen and nutrients from the placenta to the baby, which in turn will lead to growth restriction. An ultrasound can pick up placental insufficiency. Contributing factors include high blood pressure, diabetes, blood clotting disorders, smoking, and drinking during pregnancy.

Preeclampsia

Preeclampsia will be discussed in more detail below but is potentially linked to issues regarding the placenta.

Placenta Previa

This is when the placenta partially or completely blocks the cervix, causing an obstruction that the baby can't pass through during vaginal delivery, meaning C-section is necessary. The cause is as of yet unknown.

Placenta Abruption

Placenta abruption is potentially life-threatening to the mother and the baby and is when the placenta tears away from the uterine wall before the baby is born. This can cause preterm birth, or even stillbirth, as the placenta is what provides oxygen and nutrients to the baby. Excessive bleeding caused by placenta abruption is incredibly dangerous to the mother (and in turn the baby), as this can lead to a loss of consciousness, hypovolemic shock, organ failure, and other complications.

Factors that can increase the risk of placenta abruption are high blood pressure, pregnancy over 40, infection of the uterus, smoking, and substance abuse.

Placenta Accreta

On the opposite end of placenta abruption, is Placenta Accreta, as this is a condition where the placenta is too attached to the uterine wall. It's not really an issue until after birth when the placenta must be delivered to prevent necrosis and infection. It will have to be removed by a doctor, or in severe cases, be treated with a hysterectomy.

Placenta Increta is when the placenta invades the uterine muscles, whereas Placenta Percreta is when the placenta grows past the uterus's walls. These have to be corrected surgically.

Preeclampsia

Preeclampsia is serious and life-threatening to you and your baby. The most identifying characteristics of preeclampsia are high blood pressure (higher than 140/90 mmHg), and high levels of protein in the urine. This in turn leads to heart and organ complications, such as damage and dysfunction due to insufficient blood and oxygen supply. Protein in your urine is an indication of kidney problems.

Risk factors for developing preeclampsia:

- pre-existing high blood pressure
- family history of preeclampsia
- obesity
- diabetes
- autoimmune conditions (for example lupus)
- expecting more than one baby

Other signs and symptoms of preeclampsia include:

- headaches
- visual disturbances
- swelling of hands and face
- shortness of breath
- pain on the right side of the abdomen

Dangerous symptoms that require hospitalization:

- hypertensive crisis (160/110 mmHg)
- liver and kidney dysfunction
- fluid in the lungs
- thrombocytopenia (low blood platelet count)

The cause of preeclampsia is unclear, and the onset is usually around week 37, near the due date. It can happen earlier and can lead to preterm birth.

If you're diagnosed with pre-eclampsia, your baby might need to be delivered via C-section for your and your baby's safety. This will depend on the severity. Additional treatment depends on the severity of your case as well, and the preferences of your practitioner, and you will be closely monitored. Magnesium sulfate is likely to be administered during labor and following delivery for 24 hours to prevent eclampsia.

A healthy lifestyle (exercise, healthy, diet, and healthy weight) is all recommended to lower the chance of developing pre-eclampsia.

Eclampsia

Eclampsia is a complication of pre-eclampsia where the blood pressure rises so high, that it causes violent seizures. It can also lead to unconsciousness and agitation. At this point, the patient will be treated with anticonvulsants, epilepsy medication, and possibly steroids to help the baby's lungs mature for early delivery.

Eclampsia has a high risk of death for you and/or your baby and medical intervention is essential.

Premature Rupture of Membranes (PROM)

In rare cases, a mother's water may break before week 34, which can cause preterm labor and preterm birth, or can cause infections to develop. In these cases, the woman will have to be monitored at the hospital.

Reasons for PROM include:

- Infections of the uterus
- Using dangerous and illicit substances while pregnant
- Family history of PROM
- Being underweight and having poor nutrition
- Short cervical length
- Smoking during pregnancy

Complications During and After Labor

Not Going into Labor Naturally, and Labor not Progressing

In both cases, induction is usually employed unless the practitioner decides on alternative interventions (such as a C-section). Methods and reasons for inducing labor were discussed in *Delivery Time* under *Did You Need Induction?* but to recap, labor is induced when:

- the baby is overdue
- the mother is diabetic
- the mother has high blood pressure
- the mother or the baby has other health complications that make it necessary
- the baby is growing too slowly
- the mother's water broke and there are no contractions within 24 hours
- contractions are irregular, or not strong enough, or not frequent enough
- if any part of the labor process is starting to take too long according to the practitioner
- oligohydramnios
- infection in the uterus
- premature rupture of membranes

Perineal Tears

During delivery, there's a chance for the vagina or any of the surrounding tissue to tear because a coconut-sized head is being pushed out through the birth canal after all, and sometimes that head can be a bit too big, or the vagina can't stretch far enough. More serious tears will be closed up with stitches, but they usually heal on their own.

Umbilical Cord Complications

As mentioned previously in *Delivery Time*, there's a chance that the umbilical cord can get caught on the way out of the birth canal, or can even wrap around the baby's neck. The cord can also exit the birth canal ahead of the baby, a condition known as umbilical cord prolapse. The practitioner has to intervene to prevent the baby from asphyxiating; this is a medical emergency and will likely proceed to C-section.

Possible causes for umbilical cord prolapse:

- Preterm labor
- PROM
- Expecting multiples
- Polyhydramnios
- Breech presentation

A longer umbilical cord (longer than 100 cm) is more likely to knot, prolapse, or get entangled. Short umbilical cords (shorter than 30 cm) can delay labor, and cause placental abruption, cord rupture, or inversion of the baby.

Abnormal Fetal Heart Rate

The baby's heart rate is monitored throughout labor, especially if labor was induced. If at any point the baby's heart rate becomes concerning, possibly indicating distress, the practitioner may have to conduct an emergency C-section to get the baby out as quickly as possible.

Shoulder Dystocia

Shoulder Dystocia occurs when the baby's shoulder gets stuck as it exits the birth canal, and the head is already out. There isn't really a way to predict or prevent shoulder dystocia from happening. Having a smaller pelvis, or having a large baby, could be contributing factors.

This is considered a medical emergency, as injury to the baby and to the mother needs to be prevented while delivery also needs to happen as fast as possible. The practitioner may consider an episiotomy or C-section. The steps normally followed are HELPERR:

- H - Help: The practitioner will immediately call for additional assistance.
- E - Evaluate for episiotomy: An episiotomy will be considered if necessary for additional movement room.
- L - Legs: The practitioner may ask you to pull your thighs up to your belly to flatten out the pelvis. This is also known as the McRoberts maneuver.
- P - Pressure: The practitioner will ask the nurse to apply pressure to the lower abdomen/above the pubic bone and attempt to rotate the baby's shoulder free. This is called supra-pubic pressure.
- E - Enter maneuvers: The practitioner may try to rotate and manipulate the baby inside the vagina.
- R - Remove posterior arm: The practitioner may try to use Jacquemier's maneuver, where they will pull out one of the baby's arms to hopefully make it easier for the shoulder to come out.

- R - Roll the patient: The practitioner may request the mother to change positions and turn over onto their hands and knees, also known as the Gaskin maneuver.

In severe cases, the practitioner may break the baby's clavicle to help them out. They may also push the baby back into the uterus (Zavanelli maneuver) and proceed to C-section, or perform a symphysiotomy, where the cartilage of the pubic bone is cut to make the pelvic opening larger.

Risks of shoulder dystocia:

- physical injuries to the baby
- umbilical cord compression
- severe bleeding in the mother
- severe perineal tearing
- rupture of the uterus
- separation of the pubic bones
- rectovaginal fistula (an abnormal connection between the rectum and vagina)

Risk factors that may contribute to shoulder dystocia:

- diabetes and/or gestational diabetes
- unusually large baby
- expecting multiples
- abnormal pelvic structure
- obesity
- maternity age over 35

Postpartum Hemorrhage/Excessive Bleeding

If tears in the uterus occur or there are placental problems, these can cause injury and lead to heavy, often life-threatening, bleeding in the mother. This may happen during and after labor, or in rarer cases happen up to twelve weeks later. The most common cause (80% of cases) of excessive bleeding postpartum, is when the placenta is expelled but the contractions aren't strong enough to compress the arteries in the uterus, thus they continue to bleed. Blood clotting disorders can also be a causing factor.

This is considered a medical emergency, as extreme blood loss can send the mother into hypovolemic shock. Her blood pressure will drop and there will be decreased blood flow to the brain and essential organs, which can cause damage.

The treatment will depend on the cause of the bleeding.

- Tears and lacerations will be stitched and repaired.
- Any placental tissue that stayed behind will be removed.
- Contractions will be stimulated manually, or with medication.
- Tying off blood vessels to stop the bleeding.
- Using a balloon or catheter to apply pressure to the arteries in the uterus.
- Uterine artery embolization - blockers will be inserted into the arteries to stop blood flow.
- Blood transfusion to make up for lost volumes.

Our first line of defense will be an open IV with fluids, with Pitocin wide open. Remember, during induction of labor, we give very small amounts to help the uterus with contractions. After delivery, we give a lot more as we want that uterus to clamp down fast and furious to stop any bleeding that is happening. We may even opt to give an IM (intramuscular) injection of Pitocin to get that bleeding to stop. Other drugs that are preferred to help stop the bleeding are Cytotec, Methergine, and Hemabate.

Breech Presentation

Babies aren't always in the right position when labor starts, and among those complications is breech presentation. If a baby is breech, vaginal delivery is very risky, as it can cause distress to the baby, and the birth is likely to take very long. In most breech cases it's safer to opt for C-section.

- Complete breech: The baby's knees are completely bent and tucked to their chest, and their bottom is facing the birth canal.
- Incomplete breech: Only one of the baby's knees is completely bent and tucked to their chest, and their bottom is facing the birth canal.
- Frank breech: The baby is "folded" with their legs straight upward and their feet near their head; their bottom is facing the birth canal.
- Footling breech: When one or both of the baby's feet emerge first.

- Transverse lie: The baby is lying horizontally instead of vertically, and their shoulder is likely to enter the birth canal first.

Factors that increase the risk of breech presentation:

- family history of breech presentation
- expecting multiples
- preterm birth
- uterus abnormalities and/or uterine fibroids
- too much or too little amniotic fluid
- placenta previa
- a birth defect that may cause the baby not to turn into the correct position

Meconium Aspiration

Meconium is the first stool a baby passes and is usually passed after birth, but may be passed in utero in some cases. When the baby breathes in a combination of meconium and amniotic fluid, it can cause severe complications for them.

If there is meconium in the amniotic fluid, it will be stained with a dark green color.

Signs and symptoms:

- The baby's skin is bluish
- The baby is limp and unresponsive
- Breathing problems

The practitioner can diagnose meconium aspiration by checking for meconium in the amniotic fluid, listening to the baby's lungs for crackling sounds, and by taking an X-ray, which will show streaks across the baby's lungs.

The baby will be treated with antibiotics to prevent and treat possible infections. The baby will likely be put on a ventilator and artificially kept warm to maintain a healthy body temperature. Their chest can also be tapped to loosen and expel secretions.

If treated, most babies will survive. Otherwise, meconium aspiration can lead to serious infections such as pneumonia, can lead to brain and organ damage, and even death.

Complications After Birth

Postpartum Depression

A measure of low spirits, mood swings, and feeling blue after your baby's birth is normal. You're still reeling with hormones, not getting enough sleep, your baby is probably crying a lot, and your life has changed dramatically.

Some women, however, develop a more severe condition that interferes with self-care and bonding with the baby. This usually develops within a month after the baby's birth, and only lasts for a year, but can have significant consequences with regard to the mother and the baby's relationship, as well as increase the risk of developing other mental health conditions.

Symptoms include:

- restlessness
- severe anxiety
- severe depression
- insomnia
- scatterbrained and difficulty concentrating
- suicidal ideation and thoughts
- intrusive thoughts about hurting the baby
- fear of hurting the baby and not deserving to be a mother
- intense mood swings
- extreme exhaustion and fatigue
- hopelessness
- feelings of guilt and shame
- withdrawal from others

Postpartum depression affects 13 - 19% of women, and isn't something to be ashamed of. Many women don't seek out help because they're embarrassed and feel like failures. It's essential to talk to a healthcare professional if a parent (postpartum depression can affect fathers too) feels depressed, suicidal, or experiences any of the above-mentioned symptoms. Postpartum depression can be treated and it's very important that the affected parent get the support and help they need.

There are some risk factors that can make a parent more likely to develop postpartum depression. Namely:

- pre-existing depression and or anxiety disorder
- family history of postpartum depression, or other mental health disorders
- lack of support during and after pregnancy
- low self-esteem
- stressful and major life events (such as the death of a loved one, or an accident)
- poor relationship with your partner
- financial stress
- being a single parent
- unwanted or unexpected pregnancy
- having a baby with difficult needs (such as a baby born with a genetic or developmental disorder)

Postpartum depression can be treated with both therapy and medication. Therapy usually involves cognitive behavioral therapy (CBT) or interpersonal psychotherapy (IPT). The most common medication prescribed for postpartum depression, which also shows improvement of symptoms in most people, includes SSRIs such as fluoxetine.

Mothers can breastfeed while taking fluoxetine, but the risk-benefit of breastfeeding while taking antidepressants should be evaluated for each individual by their prescriber.

In rare cases, 0.1 – 0.5% of cases, postpartum depression can develop into postpartum psychosis. With postpartum psychosis, the affected person can experience the following:

- hallucinations and/or delusions
- paranoia
- confusion
- obsessive thoughts about your baby
- sleep disturbances
- agitation
- may attempt to harm the baby

Postpartum psychosis is even more dangerous than postpartum depression, and it's paramount that the affected parent gets help.

Infections

Perineal or vaginal tears can lead to infections later, even with stitches, as there's a wound. Some women may also catch UTIs, kidney infections, or vaginal infections.

The following are possible signs of infection:

- fever
- swelling and redness that's warm to the touch
- pain or burning sensation when urinating
- abnormal and bad-smelling discharge
- lower back pain
- vaginal itching

It's important to catch and treat an infection early before it progresses to something more serious.

Constipation and Incontinence

Constipation after giving birth is normal and can be caused by hormones, iron supplements, and hemorrhoids. Your digestive tract needs some time to recover.

Tips for constipation:

- include more fiber in your diet
- drink lots of water and stay hydrated
- eat prunes or drink prune juice
- if all else fails, use mild laxatives

Urinary incontinence is also perfectly normal, as your muscles might still need to recover and can't quite keep everything from leaking out. Wearing pads or menstrual underwear can keep your underwear and trousers clean, but if it's serious, you can see a doctor for help.

Breast Pain and Mastitis

Whether you breastfeed or not, hormones can cause your breasts to ache and swell. Breastfeeding your baby can bring some relief, but since not all mothers can breastfeed, this can be treated with hot and cold compresses (alternate every fifteen minutes), over-the-counter pain medication, and a warm bath or shower.

Breastfeeding can bring its own discomfort as both mother and baby figure things out and find a rhythm. Lanolin cream is an excellent moisturizer for sore dry nipples as well. A lactation consultant can also help to teach you and your baby techniques that are less painful (at least until their little teeth come in).

Mastitis is a condition that can affect all mothers, whether they breastfeed or not, where (usually) one of their breasts becomes swollen and inflamed. This is generally caused by an infection of the milk ducts. Since milk is a great growth medium for bacteria, if milk "stays still" for too long, this can trigger an infection. Other ways infection can occur is if the breasts become dry and cracked, giving bacteria an entryway. Antibiotics are generally prescribed to treat mastitis. If untreated, mastitis can lead to painful abscesses.

Other signs and symptoms to look out for:

- swelling of the breast that's hot to the touch
- redness of the breast
- tenderness of the breast
- fever
- flu-like symptoms
- itching of the breast
- tenderness under your arm (and swollen glands)

Cardiovascular Disease

Otherwise known as heart disease, is the number one cause of death in women in developed countries. Whether pregnancy itself increases the risk of cardiovascular disease, or whether a pre-existing predisposition for cardiovascular disease is triggered by pregnancy is as of yet unknown. Regardless, numerous risk factors can contribute to developing cardiovascular disease after giving birth:

- family history of cardiovascular disease
- high blood pressure (unrelated to pregnancy)
- preeclampsia and gestational hypertension
- obesity
- preterm labor and/or birth

The majority of women with cardiovascular disease don't present with the typical symptoms (chest pain, trouble breathing, numbness, stiff neck) and go undiagnosed and untreated. For this reason, cardiovascular screening is vital during and after pregnancy. You should immediately seek medical help if you experience any of the following:

- chest pain
- breathing difficulties
- irregular heart rate and/or regular palpitations
- seizures

Deep Vein Thrombosis

The risk for developing deep vein thrombosis (DVT) is already higher during pregnancy but is at its highest after giving birth. Hormones increase the risk of blood clotting, and a clot in the leg can cause painful swelling in the affected leg. The danger of a blood clot is if it travels to other parts of the body. If it reaches the heart or blocks blood flow to the heart, it can cause a heart attack. A clot in the lungs, called a pulmonary embolism, can also cause a heart attack, decrease oxygen levels in the body, interfere with breathing, lower blood pressure, and cause death. A blood clot in the brain can cause a stroke, which could be lethal.

Risk factors for developing DVT:

- pregnancy over the age of 35
- having given birth to three or more babies before
- family and/or personal history of DVT
- having a blood clotting condition
- a history of cardiovascular disease, lung disease, or arthritis
- severe varicose veins
- are unable to move around much, or can't use your legs (for example wheelchair users)
- obesity
- carried multiples during pregnancy
- preeclampsia
- long labor

Women who are more at risk to develop DVT after birth will likely be treated with low-molecular-weight heparin in the form of an injection that can be self-administered, which prevents blood from clotting. It's generally given to patients after certain surgeries with an increased risk of clotting as well. Other ways to prevent developing DVT are:

- staying active, alternate sitting and standing frequently
- wearing compression stockings for varicose veins
- avoiding contraception that contains estrogen in the future

Likewise, DVT is treated with heparin or other anti-clotting medication, by wearing compression stockings, and taking pain medication.

Pregnancy Loss

Loss isn't something many of us like to think about, and although it might be an unpleasant topic, it's a part of life. I would be remiss not to touch on this topic as well. I hope that you will be spared the heartache and pain of pregnancy loss. Unfortunately, many women all over the world have gone through this, even with how far medical science has come. If you've never experienced the sorrow of pregnancy loss, it's at least important to understand what others have and are going through.

Miscarriage

Pregnancy loss in the first trimester is known as an early miscarriage. Most miscarriages are early miscarriages and happen within the first ten weeks after fertilization. It doesn't matter how early the miscarriage is, however, as it can still be an emotional and difficult experience. Late miscarriage, or simply "miscarriage", is pregnancy loss between the end of the first trimester and week 20.

Causes for Miscarriage

Half of all miscarriages are caused by chromosomal abnormalities. Chromosomes are structures that carry genetic information; half are inherited from the biological father, and half are inherited from the biological mother. When a sperm fertilizes an egg cell, and one or both have an abnormal amount of chromosomes, this will lead to genetic problems with the fetus. Some genetic conditions aren't lethal, for example, Down Syndrome is due to having one extra chromosome, so the baby has 47 instead of 46. Which chromosomes are missing, or if there are extra, will determine how the fetus develops. This, unfortunately, is why not all fetuses make it past the first few weeks. Chromosomal abnormalities aren't something you can control outside of IVF, and is never your fault as genetic abnormalities can happen anytime at the cell level.

Other possible causes for early miscarriage are:

- smoking
- drinking alcohol
- abusing illicit drugs (although marijuana may be legal in some regions, it isn't safe to use during pregnancy and while breastfeeding)
- uncontrolled diabetes

- hyperthyroidism and hypothyroidism
- certain autoimmune conditions
- physical abnormalities of the uterus, such as uterine fibroids
- being underweight and malnourished
- exposure to radiation
- age (very young and older women are more at risk)
- incompetent cervix
- hormonal problems
- certain medications
- infections
- familial cardiovascular disease
- physical and/or emotional trauma
- history of previous miscarriages

Signs and Symptoms of Miscarriage

Early miscarriage:

- bleeding that starts off light and grows heavier; it might appear brown and contain clots or contain grayish tissue
- pain and cramping of the lower abdomen; it can be very painful and feel worse than menstrual cramps
- lower back pain of varying severity
- discharging large volumes of fluid from the vagina, either clear or pinkish
- symptoms of pregnancy are fading
- dizziness and faintness

Late miscarriage:

- heavy bleeding
- strong and painful abdominal cramps
- no movement from the baby
- no fetal heartbeat
- dilation of the cervix

Types of Miscarriage

Threatening Miscarriage: Some of the signs and symptoms of miscarriage are present, such as bleeding and cramping, but the cervix is closed and there is no definite sign that the pregnancy has stopped. The mother will be closely monitored, but there is a possibility that the pregnancy will continue normally and without issue.

Incomplete Miscarriage: The pregnancy is miscarrying and the embryo or fetus is no longer viable. The symptoms of miscarriage are present, but not all the pregnancy tissue has been expelled. Because some of the tissue stays behind, the woman will continue to experience cramps and bleeding. Surgery might be needed if the remaining tissue doesn't pass on its own.

Complete Miscarriage: Miscarriage symptoms were present and the embryo or fetus, along with all the pregnancy tissue, has been expelled from the body. The woman is no longer considered pregnant.

Missed Miscarriage: The embryo or fetus has passed away, but there are no signs or symptoms of miscarriage. In some cases, the body continues to produce pregnancy hormones as normal, while in other cases pregnancy symptoms stop without any other signs. This is usually picked up during the first ultrasound when no heartbeat is detected.

Septic Miscarriage: The miscarriage is caused by an infection and can be deadly to the mother. Additional symptoms include fever, chills, and a foul-smelling vaginal discharge. The mother urgently needs treatment with antibiotics, and all the infected tissue has to be removed.

Anembryonic Gestation: Fertilization and implantation happened, but the pregnancy didn't progress further.

Chemical Pregnancy: Although no fetus has formed, this is considered a type of early miscarriage where fertilization has taken place, but either implantation didn't happen, or the embryo stopped developing. The name is derived from the fact that a woman may initially test positive for pregnancy due to the presence of hCG in her urine, but later tests negative, or gets her period. Not all women who experience a chemical pregnancy realize that they've conceived and think it's a normal period. Normal pregnancies can still happen even if a woman has had a chemical pregnancy.

What To Do When a Woman Miscarries

Whether it's an incomplete miscarriage or a missed miscarriage, the woman and their practitioner will work together to decide on the best next step. Depending on how far along the pregnancy is and other factors that may impact the woman's health, the decision might be to let the miscarriage complete naturally on its own, through the aid of medication, or by removing the tissue surgically. Whatever the decision, the pregnancy tissue must be removed and the physical and emotional well-being of the woman has to come first.

<u>Non-medical Intervention:</u> The miscarriage is left to run its course on its own, and may take a few days to a few weeks, depending on the stage of the pregnancy.

<u>Medication Intervention:</u> To help the body expel all the pregnancy tissue, a woman may be given oral medication, usually misoprostol, that will trigger the uterus to contract and pass all the pregnancy tissue. This usually only takes a few days. Side effects may include cramping, nausea, and vomiting.

<u>Surgical Intervention:</u> Also known as dilation and curettage (D&C), this is a small procedure in which a practitioner dilates the cervix to remove the placenta and other pregnancy tissue from the uterus.

Ectopic Pregnancy

When the fertilized egg cell fails to pass through the fallopian tube and implants there, or anywhere outside the uterus, it's called an ectopic pregnancy and is sadly not viable. If left untreated, this can cause the fallopian tubes to rupture, and lead to fatal bleeding. That fallopian tube and the connected ovum will also no longer be functional, and decreases the woman's future chance of ovulation and thus fertility.

Not all ectopic pregnancies have a specific cause, but some cases have been caused by the following:

- scarring and/or physical abnormalities of the fallopian tubes
- hormonal factors
- certain genetic conditions
- birth defects

A woman's risk for an ectopic pregnancy also increases with the following:

- maternity age over 35
- history of pelvic surgeries and/or complications
- endometriosis
- previous ectopic pregnancies
- conception via IUD
- use of fertility medication to produce multiple egg cells
- smoking
- STIs

The symptoms of an ectopic pregnancy are:

- sharp pain and cramping on one side of the lower abdomen or pelvic area
- light spotting or bleeding (initially)
- rectal pressure
- dizziness and feeling faint

An ectopic pregnancy is confirmed with ultrasound and blood tests, and its paramount that it be discovered early to prevent any serious problems to the woman's health and to possibly save the fallopian tube in question. An ectopic pregnancy is either treated surgically (via laparoscopy) or treated with medication such as methotrexate. The woman will be monitored afterward to ensure that all the pregnancy tissue has indeed been expelled.

Molar Pregnancy

Sometimes all the signs and symptoms are there, but unfortunately, no baby is developing inside. This can be incredibly disappointing, particularly if a woman has been very excited to become pregnant, or has been struggling to become pregnant.

It also starts with a fertilized egg, but instead of developing into a fetus, a mass of cysts forms out of the placenta. The woman may experience dark brown or bright red bleeding, severe nausea and vomiting, and in some cases severe cramping.

Signs that a practitioner looks for include:

- high blood pressure
- a doughy uterus instead of a firm uterus
- an unusually large uterus
- no presence of a viable fetus or embryo
- unusually high levels of thyroid hormone

If a molar pregnancy is diagnosed, it has to be treated with D&C, and the woman needs to be monitored afterward to make sure cancer doesn't develop. Fortunately, molar pregnancies are incredibly rare. Maternity age over 35 and a history of multiple miscarriages increases the risk of a molar pregnancy.

Stillbirth

Pregnancy loss after week 20, or losing a baby during labor or birth, is called a stillbirth. This is heartbreaking to experience and can be traumatic. A baby can be stillborn due to:

- birth defects
- problems with the placenta
- problems with the umbilical cord
- poor fetal development
- health conditions of the mother, such as diabetes,
- preeclampsia
- infection
- severe trauma

A lack of movement from the baby and no heartbeat are usually the only signs that the baby has passed while still in the uterus. Usually, the woman will have to wait for labor to start naturally, or labor will be induced. A C-section will be done in emergencies, or if the mom and practitioner feel it's the best course of action.

Stillbirths can't always be prevented, but the following can improve a woman's chances of avoiding the risk:

- avoiding smoking, alcohol, and recreational substances
- monitoring and being aware of the baby's movement
- going for regularly scheduled consultations with a practitioner
- managing a healthy weight before and during pregnancy
- avoiding infections where possible
- reporting any bleeding and pain to the practitioner, or any concerning symptoms
- avoiding raw meat and make sure all meat is thoroughly cooked
- getting the flu vaccine
- taking supplements as recommended
- avoiding caffeine

A woman's risk for stillbirth is also increased in the following cases:

- expecting multiples
- maternity age over 35

- obesity
- health conditions such as diabetes and heart conditions
- malnutrition

What happens after the stillborn baby is born is up to the parents. They may want to hold the baby or take a memento home. It's a personal issue and is entirely their decision. The practitioner will offer to conduct tests to possibly determine the cause. These include blood tests, infection tests, thyroid function tests, genetic tests, and physical examinations, particularly of the umbilical cord and placenta. They may also ask for permission to conduct a post-mortem, an in-depth examination of the baby.

Breast Milk After Stillbirth

The body may still produce breast milk after stillbirth, as the hormonal process for lactation has already been set in motion. This can be devastating to experience on top of going through loss. Mothers can choose to let the milk dry out on its own, or can take medication to stop milk production. Dopamine agonists are prescribed to counter milk production but are contraindicated for women with preeclampsia. It's up to the mother what she is most comfortable with and provides the best closure.

What To Do After Experiencing Loss

Miscarriage and stillbirth are traumatic experiences. It's important for those involved, particularly the mother, to get the help and support they need to recover. This not only refers to physical care but emotional and psychological care as well. The parents may experience guilt, depression, or severe anxiety over what happened, and may develop PTSD. This can negatively impact possible future pregnancies, as well as other areas of their life.

Counseling and Therapy

Some religions have trained counselors that can help parents through the healing process based on their personal beliefs, usually for free. This can provide comfort to some as they find strength and support in their faith and from their religious community.

There are also many trained therapists and psychologists who specialize in bereavement. They allow the parents to express their emotions and grief without judgment and can teach them healthy coping mechanisms and strategies to recover.

If a counselor, therapist, psychologist, or other mental health care provider doesn't suit a person's needs, there's no obligation to continue seeing them. Everyone is different, and everyone needs a different type of support.

Important To Keep in Mind

Not everyone will understand what someone who is grieving is going through, and this may unintentionally lead to some hurtful comments and words when they need support. If people have trouble understanding, tell them exactly what you need, whether you need help with cooking, taking the dog for a walk, or with the laundry.

Try asking for a few days off from work. Not all employers are empathetic and understanding, but hopefully, you'll be given the time you need.

Breaking the same horrible news over and over is difficult. If you're not up to it, ask someone willing to help pass on the news to whomever you wish. It's recommended that your employer and key colleagues know if only to give you the space and respect you need. You can also pass along any requests, such as no posting about it on social media, when you're ready to see people, among other things.

Your feelings are valid. Cry when you need to cry, be angry when you feel angry. Don't suppress your emotions. If you're out in public and are embarrassed, go have a good cry in the public bathroom. Repressing emotions will only be harmful and complicate the grieving process.

Don't isolate yourself completely. For some people, it's easier to avoid the world and be alone with their grief, and some alone time is necessary, but complete isolation is unhealthy. Talk to friends and or family, and if they're unsupportive, there are numerous support groups online as well as therapy.

Take care of your needs, and take things one step at a time. Feeling too overwhelmed to do all the chores? Then don't do it.

Just make sure you stay fed, hydrated, and clean. Sleep is also vital. If you have trouble falling asleep, try to find techniques that work for you, or listen to a calming podcast or audiobook. Sleeping too much is also unhealthy. If you feel like you have trouble dragging yourself out of bed, try to find distractions that don't take up all your energy, such as watching your favorite comfort movie.

Don't blame yourself or your partner. Even if you tried everything in your power, sometimes bad things happen for no reason at all. You or your partner aren't bad people who caused this thing to happen. This way of thinking will only hurt and make it more difficult to heal. Don't deny feelings of guilt completely, recognize them for what they are, and then dismiss them as lies. It's easier said than done but becomes easier with practice.

Journal. Write down all your thoughts and feelings in a notebook. You don't have to read anything back if you don't want to. This also helps to process what's going on inside and can transfer some of that hurt onto the page.

Don't give up. It hurts, and it feels like you'll never recover. Take your time to recover, but also know that one day you will be able to get up and make breakfast again. Things won't go back to the way they were, but you can learn to live life in a new way. Don't feel guilty when you find joy in something again. Moving on isn't forgetting.

If you want to try again, wait until you're one hundred percent physically, emotionally, and mentally ready. If you have a partner, keep in mind their needs as well. It has to be your choice and your choice alone. No one should force you to do it, and no one should talk you out of it either (unless your practitioner heavily advises against it for your health).

Conclusion

Thank you for letting me accompany you on this exciting journey of yours! Hopefully, you not only feel prepared but also reassured after reading through this book. There are some interesting statistics on how much the average woman in the US knows about her own body, as well as what to expect when she's pregnant. As long as you read through pretty much everything in the previous chapters, most (if not all) of your questions should be answered!

As you've seen, there's a lot that happens during pregnancy; your body goes through many dramatic changes. Fortunately, the vast majority of pregnancies and deliveries proceed without complications and lead to healthy babies. 83% of babies born in the US are breastfeeding and healthy when discharged.

And even if there are complications, as long as you regularly see your healthcare practitioner, most issues can be treated or handled safely. With the technology and knowledge at the disposal of healthcare professionals, most serious conditions can be prevented as long as the correct steps are taken before and during pregnancy.

The most important to take from this book, however, is that you take responsibility for your health. This includes every aspect of your well-being, not just your physical health, but also your mental health. Most problems related to becoming pregnant, pregnancy, labor, and delivery, are due to lifestyle choices. If all of that's in place, trust in your practitioner to take things from there and try to enjoy the experience!

My hope for you is that your pregnancy will be an uncomplicated, interesting, and wonderful experience, that labor will go smoothly, and that you will deliver a happy, healthy, bundle of joy!

I hope to see you soon in *First-Time Parents: A Clear Guide and How-To for All Things Baby Birth - 1 Month.*

If you enjoyed this book, would you be so kind as to go back and leave a review? This will allow many others a better chance at seeing and purchasing the book. Thank you.

References

Akang, E., Oremosu, A., Osinubi, A., James, A., Biose, I., Dike, S., & Idoko, K. (2017). Alcohol-induced male infertility: Is sperm DNA fragmentation a causative?. *Journal of Experimental and Clinical Anatomy, 16*(1), 53-53.

Anderson, B. (2021, January 11). *Beyond "near me": How to find the best OB-GYN for you*. HealthPartners Blog. https://www.healthpartners.com/blog/insider-tips-for-finding-the-right-ob-gyn-for-you/

Anonymous. (2020, August 13). *17 Natural Ways to Boost Fertility*. Healthline. https://www.healthline.com/nutrition/16-fertility-tips-to-get-pregnant#Takeaway

Anonymous. (n.d.). How does mumps affect male fertility? | NOVA IVF. Www.novaivffertility.com. Retrieved September 20, 2022, from https://www.novaivffertility.com/fertility-help/how-does-mumps-affect-male-fertility

Anonymous. (n.d.). *Male Fertility Drugs*. Healthcare.utah.edu. https://healthcare.utah.edu/fertility/treatments/male-fertility-drugs.php

Anonymous. (2021, March 4). *Iron in pregnancy* | Tommy's. Www.tommys.org. https://www.tommys.org/pregnancy-information/im-pregnant/nutrition-in-pregnancy/iron-pregnancy

Anonymous. (2022, July 21). *How Long Does Morning Sickness Last? Plus, Tips for Relief.* Healthline. https://www.healthline.com/health/pregnancy/how-long-does-morning-sickness-last

Anonymous. (2021, November 1). Pregnancy Hemorrhoids: Causes, Risks, Treatment. Healthline. https://www.healthline.com/health/pregnancy/pregnancy-hemorrhoids#prevention

Anonymous. (2020, February 27). *How to Prepare for Labor Induction: What to Expect and What to Ask*. Healthline. https://www.healthline.com/health/pregnancy/how-to-prepare-for-labor-induction#takeaway

Anonymous. (2016, March 29). *Management of Labor.* Healthline. https://www.healthline.com/health/pregnancy/management-labor

Anonymous. (2018, July 17). *Hyperemesis Gravidarum: Causes, Symptoms, and Diagnosis.* Healthline. https://www.healthline.com/health/hyperemesis-gravidarum

Anonymous. (2018, September 12). *Eclampsia: Causes, Symptoms, and Diagnosis*. Healthline. https://www.healthline.com/health/eclampsia#:~:text=What%20is%20eclampsia%3F

Anonymous. (2017, January 9). *What are some common complications during labor and delivery?* Https://Www.nichd.nih.gov/. https://www.nichd.nih.gov/health/topics/labor-delivery/topicinfo/complications#

Anonymous. (2019, August 27). *Common Postpartum Complications, Plus When to See a Doctor.* Healthline. https://www.healthline.com/health/pregnancy/postpartum-complications#excessive-bleeding

Anonymous. (2020, October). *Hepatitis B Foundation: Pregnancy and Hepatitis B*. Www.hepb.org. https://www.hepb.org/treatment-and-management/pregnancy-and-hbv/

Anonymous. (2019). *Pregnant women and influenza - Influenza.* Nsw.gov.au. https://www.health.nsw.gov.au/Infectious/Influenza/Pages/influenza_and_pregnancy.aspx#:~:text=Flu%20is%20serious%20for%20pregnant%20women%20and%20their%20babies

Anonymous. (2022, May 17). *Yeast Infections and Pregnancy: Causes, Symptoms & More.* Healthline. https://www.healthline.com/health/pregnancy/candidias-yeast-infection#complications

Aye, C. Y., Boardman, H., & Leeson, P. (2017). Cardiac disease after pregnancy: a growing problem. *European Cardiology Review, 12*(1), 20.

Bai, S., Wan, Y., Zong, L., Li, W., Xu, X., Zhao, Y., ... & Guo, T. (2020). Association of alcohol intake and semen parameters in men with primary and secondary infertility: a cross-sectional study. *Frontiers in physiology, 11*, 566625.

Balkawade, N. U., & Shinde, M. A. (2012). Study of length of umbilical cord and fetal outcome: a study of 1,000 deliveries. *The Journal of Obstetrics and Gynecology of India, 62*(5), 520-525.

Besich, B. (2021, November 2). *Water Birth: Pros, Cons, and What You Need to Know*. Parents. https://www.parents.com/pregnancy/giving-birth/vaginal/what-is-water-birth/

Best, D. & Bhattacharya, S. (2015). Obesity and fertility. *Hormone Molecular Biology and Clinical Investigation, 24*(1), 5-10. https://doi.org/10.1515/hmbci-2015-0023

Bly, K. C., Ellis, S. A., Ritter, R. J., & Kantrowitz-Gordon, I. (2020). A survey of midwives' attitudes toward men in midwifery. *Journal of midwifery & women's health, 65*(2), 199-207.

Brusie, C. (2017, January 8). *UTI During Pregnancy: How to Treat.* Healthline. https://www.healthline.com/health/pregnancy/treat-a-uti

Buck, K. S., & Littleton, H. L. (2013). Stereotyped beliefs about male and female OB-GYNS: relationship to provider choice and patient satisfaction. *Journal of Psychosomatic Obstetrics & Gynecology, 35*(1), 1–7. https://doi.org/10.3109/0167482x.2013.866646

Bulletti, C., Coccia, M. E., Battistoni, S., & Borini, A. (2010). Endometriosis and infertility. *Journal of assisted reproduction and genetics, 27*(8), 441-447.

Cafasso, J. (2014, October 2). *Complications During Pregnancy and Delivery.* Healthline; Healthline Media. https://www.healthline.com/health/pregnancy/delivery-complications#complications

Cantineau, A. E., Janssen, M. J., Cohlen, B. J., & Allersma, T. (2014). Synchronised approach for intrauterine insemination in subfertile couples. *Cochrane Database of Systematic Reviews,* (12).

Carneiro, M. M. (2014). What is the role of hysteroscopic surgery in the management of female infertility? A review of the literature. *Surgery Research and Practice,* 2014.

Chua, S. J., Akande, V. A., & Mol, B. W. J. (2017). Surgery for tubal infertility. *Cochrane Database of Systematic Reviews,* (1).

Cleveland Clinic. (2021, March 30). *Craniosynostosis: Symptoms, Diagnosis, Treatment. Cleveland Clinic.* https://my.clevelandclinic.org/health/articles/6000-craniosynostosis#:~:text=The%20sutures%20of%20the%20skull

Cleveland Clinic. (2020, April 3). *Positions Of Baby In Womb.* Cleveland Clinic. https://my.clevelandclinic.org/health/articles/9677-fetal-positions-for-birth#:~:text=Ideally

Cleveland Clinic. (2022, February 16). *Labor & Delivery: Signs, Progression & What To Expect.* Cleveland Clinic. https://my.clevelandclinic.org/health/articles/9676-labor-delivery#:~:text=The%20average%20labor%20lasts%2012%20for%20labor%2C%20the%20baby

Cleveland Clinic. (2022, April 29). *Electronic Fetal Monitoring: Purpose, Procedure & Results.* Cleveland Clinic. https://my.clevelandclinic.org/health/diagnostics/22940-electronic-fetal-monitoring

Cleveland Clinic. (2022, Summer 8). *C-Section (Cesarean Birth): Procedure & Risks*. Cleveland Clinic. https://my.clevelandclinic.org/health/treatments/7246-cesarean-birth-c-section

Cleveland Clinic. (2021, October 7). *Breech Baby: Causes, Complications, Turning & Delivery.* Cleveland Clinic. https://my.clevelandclinic.org/health/diseases/21848-breech-baby

Cleveland Clinic. (2019, July 22). *Miscarriage: Risks, Symptoms, Causes & Treatments.* Cleveland Clinic. https://my.clevelandclinic.org/health/diseases/9688-miscarriage

Cleveland Clinic. (2021, December 11). *Chemical Pregnancy: Causes, Symptoms & Treatment.* Cleveland Clinic. https://my.clevelandclinic.org/health/diseases/22188-chemical-pregnancy

Cleveland Clinic. (2021, December 14). *Oligohydramnios: Causes, Symptoms, Diagnosis & Treatment.* Cleveland Clinic. https://my.clevelandclinic.org/health/diseases/22179-oligohydramnios#:~:text=Oligohydramnios%20is%20when%20you%20have

Cleveland Clinic. (2022, May 15). *Amnioinfusion: Purpose, Procedure, Results & Risks.* Cleveland Clinic. https://my.clevelandclinic.org/health/treatments/23268-amnioinfusion

Cleveland Clinic. (2020, December 20). *Multiple Birth: Twins, Triplets, Complications & Symptoms.* Cleveland Clinic. https://my.clevelandclinic.org/health/articles/9710-expecting-twins-or-triplets#:~:text=A%20multiple%20pregnancy%20is%20a

Cleveland Clinic. (2014). *Umbilical Cord Prolapse Causes, Management & More | Cleveland Clinic.* Cleveland Clinic. https://my.clevelandclinic.org/health/diseases/12345-umbilical-cord-prolapse

Cleveland Clinic. (2022, January 23). *Shoulder Dystocia: Signs, Causes, Prevention & Complications.* Cleveland Clinic. https://my.clevelandclinic.org/health/diseases/22311-shoulder-dystocia

Cleveland Clinic. (2022, January 3). P*ostpartum Hemorrhage: Causes, Risks, Diagnosis & Treatment*. Cleveland Clinic. https://my.clevelandclinic.org/health/diseases/22228-postpartum-hemorrhage

De Ziegler, D., Borghese, B., & Chapron, C. (2010). Endometriosis and infertility: pathophysiology and management. *The Lancet, 376*(9742), 730-738.

Ding, G. L., Liu, Y., Liu, M. E., Pan, J. X., Guo, M. X., Sheng, J. Z., & Huang, H. F. (2015). The effects of diabetes on male fertility and epigenetic regulation during spermatogenesis. *Asian journal of andrology, 17*(6), 948.

Dormuth, C. R., Winquist, B., Fisher, A., Wu, F., Reynier, P., Suissa, S., ... & Paterson, J. M. (2021). Comparison of pregnancy outcomes of patients treated with ondansetron vs alternative antiemetic medications in a multinational, population-based cohort. *JAMA network open, 4*(4), e215329-e215329.

Elflein, J. (2022, May 20). *Mothers medical or health characteristics U.S. 2020*. Statista. https://www.statista.com/statistics/276087/medical-or-health-characteristics-of-births-for-us-mothers/

Elflein, J. (2021, June 10). *Women's knowledge gap about their reproductive system U.S*. 2020. Statista. https://www.statista.com/statistics/1242775/us-women-s-knowledge-gap-about-reproductive-system/

Erdal, H., Holst, L., Heitmann, K., & Trovik, J. (2022). Antiemetic treatment of hyperemesis gravidarum in 1,064 Norwegian women and the impact of European warning on metoclopramide: a retrospective cohort study 2002–2019. *BMC Pregnancy and Childbirth, 22*(1), 1-13.

Ernst-Milner, S. (2018, November 13). *The TAPS Support Foundation - What Is TAPS In Twins?* TAPS Support. https://www.tapssupport.com/what-is-taps-in-twins/

Feedspot Media Database Team. (2020, July 21). *Top 15 Pregnancy Forums, Discussion and Message Boards in 2022.* Feedspot Blog. https://blog.feedspot.com/pregnancy_forums/

Gadalla, M. A., Norman, R. J., Tay, C. T., Hiam, D. S., Melder, A., Pundir, J., ... & Moran, L. J. (2020). Medical and surgical treatment of reproductive outcomes in polycystic ovary syndrome: an overview of systematic reviews. *International journal of fertility & sterility, 13*(4), 257.

Gude, D. (2012). Alcohol and fertility. *Journal of human reproductive sciences, 5*(2), 226.

Habel, C., Feeley, N., Hayton, B., Bell, L., & Zelkowitz, P. (2015). Causes of women' s postpartum depression symptoms: Men' s and women' s perceptions. *Midwifery, 31*(7), 728-734.

Harris, N. (2019, January 22). *6 Things You Didn't Know About Home Birth.* Parents; Parents. https://www.parents.com/pregnancy/giving-birth/home/home-birth-facts/

Healthdirect Australia. (2021, July 21). *Cold and flu during pregnancy.* Www.pregnancybirthbaby.org.au. https://www.pregnancybirthbaby.org.au/cold-and-flu-during-pregnancy#:~:text=If%20you%20have%20flu%20while

Healthline Medical Network. (2012, March 15). *Infections in Pregnancy: Bacterial Vaginosis.* Healthline; Healthline Media. https://www.healthline.com/health/pregnancy/infections-bacterial-vaginosis

Hirsch, L. (2014). *Intrauterine Growth Restriction (IUGR) (for Parents) - KidsHealth.* Kidshealth.org. https://kidshealth.org/en/parents/iugr.html

Jie, L., Li, D., Yang, C., & Haiying, Z. (2018). Tamoxifen versus clomiphene citrate for ovulation induction in infertile women. *European Journal of Obstetrics & Gynecology and Reproductive Biology, 228*, 57-64.

Johnson, N. P. (2014). Metformin use in women with polycystic ovary syndrome. *Annals of translational medicine, 2*(6).

Lebbi, I., Ben Temime, R., Fadhlaoui, A., & Feki, A. (2015). Ovarian drilling in PCOS: is it really useful?. *Frontiers in surgery, 2*, 30.

Livshits, A., & Seidman, D. S. (2009). Fertility issues in women with diabetes. *Women's Health, 5*(6), 701-707.

Lord, M., Marino, S., & Kole, M. (2022). *Amniotic Fluid Index.* PubMed; StatPearls Publishing. https://www.ncbi.nlm.nih.gov/books/NBK441881/#:~:text=A%20normal%20amniotic%20fluid%20index

Marcin, A. (2017, April 27). *Natural Ways to Induce Labor.* Healthline; Healthline Media. https://www.healthline.com/health/pregnancy/natural-ways-to-induce-labor

Marple, K. (2021). Giving birth: *What to pack in your hospital bag | BabyCenter*. BabyCenter. https://www.babycenter.com/pregnancy/your-body/packing-for-the-hospital-or-birth-center_185

Martinez, L., Zieve, D., & Conaway, B. (2020, March 12). *Breech - series—Types of breech presentation: MedlinePlus Medical Encyclopedia*. Medlineplus.gov. https://medlineplus.gov/ency/presentations/100193_3.htm#:~:text=There%20are%20three%20types%20of

Mayo Clinic. (2019, June 22). *In vitro fertilization (IVF) - Mayo Clinic*. Mayoclinic.org; Mayo Foundation for Medical Education and Research. https://www.mayoclinic.org/tests-procedures/in-vitro-fertilization/about/pac-20384716

Mayo Clinic. (2018). *Can lifestyle choices boost my chance of getting pregnant?* Mayo Clinic. https://www.mayoclinic.org/healthy-lifestyle/getting-pregnant/in-depth/female-fertility/art-20045887

Mayo Clinic. (2022, August 6). Prenatal care: 1st trimester visits. Mayo Clinic. https://www.mayoclinic.org/healthy-lifestyle/pregnancy-week-by-week/in-depth/prenatal-care/art-20044882#:~:text=Your%20health%20care%20provider%20might%20do%20a%20physical%20exam%2C%20including

Mayo Clinic. (2020, August 25). *Prenatal testing: Is it right for you?* Mayo Clinic. https://www.mayoclinic.org/healthy-lifestyle/pregnancy-week-by-week/in-depth/prenatal-testing/art-20045177

Mayo Clinic. (2017). *First trimester pregnancy: What to expect.* Mayo Clinic. https://www.mayoclinic.org/healthy-lifestyle/pregnancy-week-by-week/in-depth/pregnancy/art-20047208

Mayo Clinic. (2017). *Second trimester pregnancy: What to expect.* Mayo Clinic. https://www.mayoclinic.org/healthy-lifestyle/pregnancy-week-by-week/in-depth/pregnancy/art-20047732

Mayo Clinic. (2020, August 26). *Gestational diabetes - Symptoms and causes.* Mayo Clinic. https://www.mayoclinic.org/diseases-conditions/gestational-diabetes/symptoms-causes/syc-20355339#:~:text=Gestational%20diabetes%20is%20diabetes%20diagnosed

Mayo Clinic. (2018). *Incompetent cervix - Symptoms and causes.* Mayo Clinic. https://www.mayoclinic.org/diseases-conditions/incompetent-cervix/symptoms-causes/syc-20373836

Mayo Clinic. (2018). *Home birth: Know the pros and cons.* Mayo Clinic. https://www.mayoclinic.org/healthy-lifestyle/labor-and-delivery/in-depth/home-birth/art-20046878

Mayo Clinic. (2018). *Preterm labor - Symptoms and causes.* Mayo Clinic. https://www.mayoclinic.org/diseases-conditions/preterm-labor/symptoms-causes/syc-20376842

Mayo Clinic. (2018, September 1). *Postpartum depression - Symptoms and Causes.* Mayo Clinic. https://www.mayoclinic.org/diseases-conditions/postpartum-depression/symptoms-causes/syc-20376617

Mayo Clinic. (2019). *Water breaking: Understand this sign of labor.* Mayo Clinic. https://www.mayoclinic.org/healthy-lifestyle/labor-and-delivery/in-depth/water-breaking/art-20044142

Mayo clinic. (2017). *Cytomegalovirus (CMV) infection - Symptoms and causes.* Mayo Clinic. https://www.mayoclinic.org/diseases-conditions/cmv/symptoms-causes/syc-20355358

Mayo Clinic. (2020). *Hepatitis B - Symptoms and causes.* Mayo Clinic. https://www.mayoclinic.org/diseases-conditions/hepatitis-b/symptoms-causes/syc-20366802

Mayo Clinic. (2020, October 13). *Toxoplasmosis - Diagnosis and treatment - Mayo Clinic.* Www.mayoclinic.org. https://www.mayoclinic.org/diseases-conditions/toxoplasmosis/diagnosis-treatment/drc-20356255#:~:text=Spiramycin%20is%20routinely%20used%20to

Mayo Clinic. (2021, March 19). *Laser therapy for twin-twin transfusion syndrome offers best outcomes - Mayo Clinic.* Www.mayoclinic.org. https://www.mayoclinic.org/medical-professionals/obstetrics-gynecology/news/laser-therapy-for-twin-twin-transfusion-syndrome-offers-best-outcomes/mac-20509521#:~:text=Twin%2Dtwin%20transfusion%20syndrome%20can

Mayo Clinic. (2018). *Conjoined twins - Symptoms and causes.* Mayo Clinic. https://www.mayoclinic.org/diseases-conditions/conjoined-twins/symptoms-causes/syc-20353910

Mazur, D. J., & Lipshultz, L. I. (2018). Infertility in the aging male. *Current Urology Reports, 19*(7), 1-9.

Meconium Aspiration Syndrome. (n.d.). Www.hopkinsmedicine.org. https://www.hopkinsmedicine.org/health/conditions-and-diseases/meconium-aspiration-syndrome#:~:text=Meconium%20aspiration%20syndrome%20occurs%20when

Metz, T. D., & Stickrath, E. H. (2015). Marijuana use in pregnancy and lactation: a review of the evidence. *American journal of obstetrics and gynecology, 213*(6), 761-778.

Mihm, M., Gangooly, S., & Muttukrishna, S. (2011). The normal menstrual cycle in women. *Animal reproduction science, 124*(3-4), 229-236.

Navabakhsh, Behrouz, Narges Mehrabi, Arezoo Estakhri, Mehdi Mohamadnejad, and Hossein Poustchi. "Hepatitis B virus infection during pregnancy: transmission and prevention." *Middle East journal of digestive diseases* 3, no. 2 (2011): 92.

NHS UK. (2018, March 6). *Mumps - Complications*. Nhs.uk. https://www.nhs.uk/conditions/mumps/complications/#:~:text=Just%20under%20half%20of%20all

NHS UK. (2020, December 2). *Doing a pregnancy test*. Nhs.uk. https://www.nhs.uk/pregnancy/trying-for-a-baby/doing-a-pregnancy-test/#:~:text=When%20you%20can%20do%20a

NHS UK. (2018, June 27). *What are the risks of group B streptococcus (GBS) infection during pregnancy?* Nhs.uk. https://www.nhs.uk/common-health-questions/pregnancy/what-are-the-risks-of-group-b-streptococcus-infection-during-pregnancy/#:~:text=Most%20pregnant%20women%20who%20carry

NHS UK. (2019). *Cytomegalovirus (CMV)*. NHS. https://www.nhs.uk/conditions/cytomegalovirus-cmv/

NHS UK. (2017, October 23). *Stillbirth - Causes*. Nhs.uk. https://www.nhs.uk/conditions/stillbirth/causes/

NHS UK. (2017, October 27). *Stillbirth - Preventing stillbirth*. Nhs.uk. https://www.nhs.uk/conditions/stillbirth/prevention/

NHS UK. (2019). *What happens if your unborn baby dies - Stillbirth*. Nhs.uk. https://www.nhs.uk/conditions/stillbirth/what-happens/

NHS UK. (2018, June 27). *What are the risks of toxoplasmosis during pregnancy?* Nhs.uk. https://www.nhs.uk/common-health-questions/pregnancy/what-are-the-risks-of-toxoplasmosis-during-pregnancy/#:~:text=Toxoplasmosis%20is%20a%20common%20infection

NHS UK. (2017, October 19). *Polyhydramnios (too much amniotic fluid).* Nhs.uk. https://www.nhs.uk/conditions/polyhydramnios/#:~:text=Polyhydramnios%20is%20where%20there%20is

Norman, R. J., Dewailly, D., Legro, R. S., & Hickey, T. E. (2007). Polycystic ovary syndrome. *The Lancet, 370*(9588), 685-697.

O'hara, M. W., & McCabe, J. E. (2013). Postpartum depression: current status and future directions. *Annual review of clinical psychology, 9*, 379-407.

Olive, D. L. (2010). Exercise and fertility: an update. *Current Opinion in Obstetrics and Gynecology, 22*(4), 259-263.

Pagán, C. N. (2021, June 8). *Getting Pregnant After Birth Control.* WebMD. https://www.webmd.com/baby/get-pregnant-after-birth-control

Pandian, Z., Gibreel, A., & Bhattacharya, S. (2015). In vitro fertilisation for unexplained subfertility. *Cochrane Database of Systematic Reviews,* (11).

Penzias, A., Bendikson, K., Butts, S., Coutifaris, C., Falcone, T., Gitlin, S., ... & Vernon, M. (2018). Smoking and infertility: a committee opinion. *Fertility and sterility, 110*(4), 611-618.

Practice Committee of the American Society for Reproductive Medicine. (2008). Smoking and infertility. *Fertility and Sterility, 90*(5), S254-S259.

Practice Committee of the American Society for Reproductive Medicine. (2014). Report on varicocele and infertility: a committee opinion. *Fertility and sterility, 102*(6), 1556-1560.

Practice Committee of the American Society for Reproductive Medicine. (2013). Use of clomiphene citrate in infertile women: a committee opinion. *Fertility and Sterility, 100*(2), 341-348.

Pritchard, J. (2016, June 17). *Mastitis | Definition and Patient Education*. Healthline. https://www.healthline.com/health/mastitis#symptoms

Purohit, P., & Vigneswaran, K. (2016). Fibroids and infertility. *Current obstetrics and gynecology reports, 5*(2), 81-88.

RCOG Patient Information Committee. (2015, April). T*reatment of venous thrombosis in pregnancy and after birth patient information leaflet.* RCOG. https://www.rcog.org.uk/for-the-public/browse-all-patient-information-leaflets/treatment-of-venous-thrombosis-in-pregnancy-and-after-birth-patient-information-leaflet/#:~:text=it%20in%20pregnancy%3F-

Riley, L. (2022, June 23). *How to Induce Labor at Home*. Parents. https://www.parents.com/pregnancy/giving-birth/labor-and-delivery/home-remedies-for-inducing-labor/

Schuppe, H. C., Pilatz, A., Hossain, H., Diemer, T., Wagenlehner, F., & Weidner, W. (2017). Urogenital infection as a risk factor for male infertility. *Deutsches Ärzteblatt International, 114*(19), 339.

Selner, M. (2018, January 8). *Ectopic Pregnancy.* Healthline; Healthline Media. https://www.healthline.com/health/pregnancy/ectopic-pregnancy

Signs of Early Miscarriage | Obstetrics & Gynecology | UC Davis Health. (n.d.). Health.ucdavis.edu. https://health.ucdavis.edu/obgyn/services/family-planning/early_miscarriage.html

Stadtmauer, L. A., Sarhan, A., Duran, E. H., Beydoun, H., Bocca, S., Pultz, B., & Oehninger, S. (2011). The impact of a gonadotropin-releasing hormone antagonist on gonadotropin ovulation induction cycles in women with polycystic ovary syndrome: a prospective randomized study. *Fertility and sterility, 95*(1), 216-220.

Starosta, A., Gordon, C. E., & Hornstein, M. D. (2020). Predictive factors for intrauterine insemination outcomes: a review. *Fertility Research and Practice, 6*(1), 1-11.

Tam, T. Y., Hill, A. M., Shatkin-Margolis, A., & Pauls, R. N. (2020). Female patient preferences regarding physician gender: a national survey. *Minerva Ginecologica, 72*(1). https://doi.org/10.23736/s0026-4784.20.04502-5

Taylor, R.B. (2011, September 22). *Using a Surrogate Mother: What You Need to Know.* WebMD; WebMD. https://www.webmd.com/infertility-and-reproduction/guide/using-surrogate-mother

Tobah, Y. B. (2021, January 6). *Yeast infection during pregnancy.* Mayo Clinic. https://www.mayoclinic.org/diseases-conditions/vaginitis/expert-answers/yeast-infection-during-pregnancy/faq-20058355#:~:text=Yeast%20infections%20are%20especially%20common

Twin Anemia Polycythemia Sequence (TAPS). (2021, August 8). Www.hopkinsmedicine.org. https://www.hopkinsmedicine.org/health/conditions-and-diseases/twin-anemia-polycythemia-sequence-taps

Twin Reversed Arterial Perfusion (TRAP). (2021, August 8). Www.hopkinsmedicine.org. https://www.hopkinsmedicine.org/health/conditions-and-diseases/twin-reversed-arterial-perfusion-trap#:~:text=Twin%20reversed%20arterial%20perfusion%20(TRAP%20sequence)%20is%20a%20rare%20condition

Twin-to-Twin Transfusion Syndrome (TTTS). (n.d.). Www.hopkinsmedicine.org. https://www.hopkinsmedicine.org/health/conditions-and-diseases/twintotwin-transfusion-syndrome-ttts#:~:text=Twin%2Dto%2Dtwin%20transfusion%20syndrome%20(TTTS)%20is%20a

Waters, D. (2022, February 10). *18 pregnancy cravings and what they mean, from chocolate to pickles.* GoodtoKnow. https://www.goodto.com/family/pregnancy/18-pregnancy-cravings-and-what-they-mean-from-chocolate-to-pickles-67916

What is Hydrops Fetalis and What Causes It? (n.d.). Children's Minnesota. https://www.childrensmn.org/services/care-specialties-departments/fetal-medicine/conditions-and-services/hydrops-fetalis/

Wild, S., & Nierenberg, C. (2018, March 27). V*aginal Birth vs. C-Section: Pros & Cons*. Live Science; Live Science. https://www.livescience.com/45681-vaginal-birth-vs-c-section.html

Yang, A. M., Cui, N., Sun, Y. F., & Hao, G. M. (2021). Letrozole for female infertility. *Frontiers in Endocrinology, 12, 737.*

Zhang, X., Zhang, J., Cai, Z., Wang, X., Lu, W., & Li, H. (2020). Effect of unilateral testicular torsion at different ages on male fertility. *Journal of International Medical Research, 48*(4), 0300060520918792.

Abbreviations

AFI: Amniotic Fluid Index

AFP: Alpha-Fetoprotein

AMA: Against Medical Advice

AMCB: American Midwifery Certification Board

AROM: Artificial Rupture of Membranes

BHA: Beta-Hydroxy Acid

BMI: Body Mass Index

BRAT: Bananas Rice Applesauce and Toast

CBT: Cognitive Behavioral Therapy

CM: Certified Midwife

CNM: Certified Nurse Midwife

CRH: Corticotropin-Releasing Hormone

C/S Cesarean Section

C-section: Cesarean Section

CVS: Chorionic Villus Sampling

D&C: Dilation and Vacuum Curettage

DVT: Deep Vein Thrombosis

EDC: Estimated Date of Confinement

EDD: Estimated Due Date

EFM: Electronic Fetal Monitor

FGR: Fetal Growth Restriction

FHR: Fetal Heart Rate

FLP: Fetoscopic Laser Photocoagulation

FSH: Follicle-Stimulating Hormone

GBS: Group Beta Streptococcus

GnRH: Gonadotropin-Releasing Hormone

HBV: Hepatitis B Virus

hCG: Human Chorionic Gonadotropin

HDN: Hemolytic Disease of the Newborn

HG: Hyperemesis Gravidarum

IUD: Intrauterine Device

IUGR: Intrauterine Growth Restriction

IUI: Intrauterine Insemination

IUPC:	Intrauterine Pressure Catheter
IV:	Intravenous Therapy
IVF:	In Vitro Fertilization
LDR:	Labor Delivery Recovery Room
LH:	Luteinizing Hormone
LOD:	Laparoscopic Ovarian Drilling
NIPT:	Non-Invasive Prenatal Testing
NST:	Non-Stress Test
NT:	Nuchal Translucency
OB:	Obstetrician
OB-GYN:	Obstetrician-Gynecologist
PCOS:	Polycystic Ovary Syndrome
PID:	Pelvic Inflammatory Disease
PROM:	Premature Rupture of Membranes
PTSD:	Post Traumatic Stress Disorder/Syndrome
PUPP:	Pruritic Urticarial Papules and Plaques
SERM:	Selective Estrogen Receptor Modulator
sFGR:	Selective Fetal Growth Restriction
SROM:	Spontaneous Rupture of Membranes

SSRIs: Selective Serotonin Reuptake Inhibitors

STD: Sexually Transmitted Disease

STIs: Sexually Transmitted Infections

SVE: Sterile Vaginal Exam

TAPS: Twin-Anemia-Polycythemia Sequence

TBA: Traditional Birth Attendant

Tdap: Tetanus, diphtheria, pertussis

TOCO: Tocodynamometer

TRAPS: Twin-Reversed-Arterial-Perfusion Syndrome

TTTS: Twin-to-Twin Transfusion Syndrome

UCs: Uterine Contractions

UTIs: Urinary Tract Infections

Glossary

ablation: The surgical destruction or removal of specific tissue, or a body part.

adipose tissue: Fatty tissue.

alveoli: Tiny air-filled structures inside the lungs responsible for the exchange of oxygen and carbon dioxide.

American Midwifery Certification Board: A regulatory body in the USA where all nurse-midwives and midwives are certified and registered.

amniocentesis: A procedure where amniotic fluid is withdrawn during pregnancy for testing.

amnioinfusion: Administration of synthetic amniotic fluid during labor.

amniotic fluid: The fluid inside the amniotic sac that protects the baby, provides nourishment, and allows them freedom of movement.

amniotic fluid index: A standardized measure of the amount of amniotic fluid in the amniotic sac.

amniotic sac: A sac filled with fluid that contains and protects the baby and the placenta during pregnancy up until birth.

amniotomy: A small hole is made in the amniotic sac to trigger the water breaking.

androgen: A hormone responsible for the development of male qualities.

anemic: A condition where there are not enough red blood cells in the body.

antibiotics: A class of medication that treats bacterial infections.

antihistamines: A class of medication that blocks the function of histamines.

aromatase inhibitor: A type of medication that blocks the function of the aromatase enzyme.

autoimmune condition: A condition where the body's immune system attacks itself.

benign: Non-cancerous

blastocyst: A structure consisting of a bundle of cells that will develop into an embryo.

bloody show: Vaginal discharge containing blood during labor.

body mass index or BMI: A value calculated from a person's height and weight that can help determine whether they are in a healthy weight range.

Braxton Hicks contractions: Small contractions during pregnancy that are not true contractions to prepare for labor in the future.

breech presentation: When a part of the baby that is not the head will exit first during vaginal delivery.

cephalic occiput anterior: The baby is positioned head downward, facing the mother's rear.

cephalic occiput posterior: The baby is positioned head downward, facing the mother's belly.

cervix: The lower structure of the uterus that forms a cylindrical canal and undergoes changes during pregnancy.

cesarean section or C/S: A surgical procedure where an incision is made in the abdomen and uterus to deliver a baby.

chorioamnionitis: A serious infection of the placenta and amniotic fluid.

colostrum: The first fluid produced by the breasts that is rich with antibodies.

constipation: The inability to defecate.

contraception: Birth control.

contraceptive implant: A device inserted under the skin, usually one of the upper arms, that steadily releases contraceptive hormones.

corpus luteum: A structure that forms inside an ovary and will start producing progesterone if implantation takes place. If implantation does not take place, it will degenerate.

corticotropin-releasing hormone: A hormone that plays a role in the stress response.

counter pressure: A technique where significant pressure is applied to an area of discomfort or pain.

cryptorchidism: A condition where one or both of the testes don't descend.

deep vein thrombosis or DVT: See page 187.

diabetes mellitus or DM: A condition characterized by insufficient insulin that causes disruptions in blood glucose levels.

diarrhea: Passing loose or liquid stool.

diastolic: The blood pressure measured in the arteries.

dichorionic-diamniotic: Each infant in a multiple pregnancy has its own placenta and its own amniotic sac.

dilation: Widening of an opening, or enlargement.

dizygotic: A type of multiple pregnancy where the babies develop from different zygotes, thus they do not look similar.

DNA: Structures in the body containing genetic material and responsible for all the cells and their functions in the body.

doula: A professional who provides emotional and practical support during pregnancy, labor, and childbirth. Doulas are not board-regulated or certified.

Down syndrome: A genetic condition where a person has one extra chromosome, causing distinct facial features, developmental problems, and heart problems.

dystocia: Slow and difficult labor and/or birth.

eclampsia: See page 172.

ectoderm: The outer layer of cells that form during the embryo's development.

ectopic pregnancy: When the zygote implants in the fallopian tubes or anywhere other than the uterus.

eczema: A skin condition where the skin becomes irritated, dry, itchy, and/or inflamed.

edema: Accumulation of fluid in the body's tissue that causes swelling.

effacement: Thinning of the uterine lining or cervix.

embryo: The first stage of a baby that forms after fertilization and implantation.

emphysema: A lung disease that causes air-filled pockets to form inside the lungs that break down the walls of the lungs and the alveoli.

encephalitis: Inflammation of the brain.

endocarditis: Inflammation of the heart.

endoderm: The innermost layer of cells that form during the embryo's development.

endometriosis: A chronic condition where the endometrium lining begins to grow outside of the uterus.

endometrium: The inner layer of the uterus that gets shed during menstruation.

epididymis: A structure in the male reproductive system where sperm are stored and mature.

epidural: A method of pain management where anesthesia is administered via an injection into the epidural space in the spinal cord.

estimated due date: An estimation of the day when labor will begin.

estradiol: See estrogen.

estrogen: The female reproductive hormone. Responsible for the development of feminine qualities and plays a role in ovulation.

fallopian tubes: A structure that forms a tube that connects the ovaries to the uterus.

false negative: When a test result comes back negative, but in reality, should be positive.

family history: If a close family member, such as parents, grandparents, or older siblings, has a certain chronic health condition, or if a certain health condition is common in the family.

fetal heart rate or FHR: The number of heart beats per minute measured from the fetus.

fetoscopic laser photocoagulation: A surgical procedure developed to treat TTTS and related conditions by ablating connections between the twins, or by functionally dividing the placenta.

fertilization: The process where a sperm fuses with an egg cell.

fetus: A baby inside the uterus.

fibroids: A condition where benign structures form inside the uterus.

flora: The microorganisms occurring inside the human body.

follicle-stimulating hormone or FSH: A naturally produced hormone that stimulates the growth of follicles in the ovary from which an egg cell will be released.

fontanelles: Flexible structures connecting the sections of the baby's skull to enable them to squeeze through the birth canal.

full term: Between week 37 and week 42 of pregnancy.

fundus: The topmost part of the uterus.

genetic disorders: Disorders due to faulty genes inherited from the parents, or due to spontaneous mutations in the genes.

genetic screening: A series of tests to determine the likelihood of the biological parents being likely to transmit a genetic disorder to the baby, as well as what type of genetic disorders.

gonadotropins: FSH and LH.

gonadotropin-releasing hormone: A naturally produced hormone responsible for the release of FSH and LH.

gonadotropin-releasing hormone antagonists: A class of medication that blocks the functioning of GnRH.

group beta streptococcus or GBS: See page 154.

hemoglobin: A protein that enables red blood cells to transport oxygen and carbon dioxide.

hemolytic disease of the newborn: See page 105.

hemophilia: A genetic condition that causes blood to clot improperly.

hemorrhage: Bleeding.

histamines: Chemicals in the body that trigger allergic symptoms.

hyperemesis gravidarum: A condition that causes excessive nausea and vomiting and requires hospitalization.

hyperinsulinemia: Abnormally high levels of insulin in the body.

hypertension: High blood pressure.

hypertensive crisis: A medical emergency where the blood pressure reading is excessively high and requires hospitalization.

hyperthyroidism: A condition where the thyroid is overactive.

hyperventilation: Abnormally fast and shallow breathing.

hypoglycemia: Abnormally low blood sugar level.

hypothyroidism: A condition where the thyroid is underactive.

hypovolemic shock: Shock induced by severe blood or other fluid loss.

hysterectomy: Permanent, surgical removal of the uterus.

implantation: The process where a fertilized egg cell attaches to the uterus wall.

immune compromised: To have a weakened immune system.

incontinence: Involuntary urination or defecation.

induction: Stimulating the uterus to start contracting to induce labor.

infertility: A condition that prevents natural reproduction.

intravenous therapy or IV: A medical practice where fluids, medication, and/or nutrients are administered directly into the patient's vein.

intrauterine device or IUD: A small device used for birth control that is inserted into the uterus.

intrauterine insemination or IUI: A process where sperm are artificially introduced into the uterus.

in vitro fertilization or IVF: A method of fertilization where the egg cell and sperm are introduced to each other outside of the body.

in utero: Inside the uterus.

jaundice: A condition that causes the skin and whites of the eyes to turn yellowish due to excess bilirubin (a pigment).

lanugo: A layer of fine, downy hair that grows and covers the fetus around week 14 of pregnancy.

laparoscopy: A surgical procedure conducted in the pelvic or abdominal areas with the help of a small camera.

leukorrhea: A thin, clear-to-white vaginal discharge to keep the cervix and vagina clean and protected.

levonorgestrel: A medication that simulates the function of progesterone.

libido: Sexual drive.

luteinizing hormone: A naturally produced hormone in the female reproductive system responsible for triggering ovulation and the development of the corpus luteum from the ovarian follicle.

malignant: Cancerous.

mastitis: Painful inflammation of the milk ducts (usually only in one breast), usually caused by an infection.

maternity age: The age at which a woman becomes pregnant.

meconium: A baby's first stool.

melasma: Tanned-looking patches of color on the skin due to hormonal changes during pregnancy.

meningitis: A condition that causes inflammation of the membranes and fluids that surround the brain and spinal cord.

menopause: The stage of a woman's life characterized by significant hormonal changes when menstruation stops and she can no longer become pregnant.

menstruation: A process that occurs once per month when the uterus lining is shed, which causes a bloody discharge for a few days from the vagina, and is often accompanied by painful cramps and moodiness. Known as a period.

mesoderm: The middle layer of cells that forms during the embryo's development.

midwife: A medical practitioner who is trained in obstetric care but cannot perform surgical interventions.

miscarriage: The death of an embryo or fetus that leads to pregnancy loss.

monochorionic-diamniotic: One placenta is shared between the infants during multiple pregnancy, but each has their own amniotic sac.

monochorionic-monoamniotic: A single placenta and a single amniotic sac is shared by all infants during multiple pregnancy.

monozygotic: A type of multiple pregnancy where all the babies have formed from a single zygote that had split, causing them to be nearly identical.

mucous plug: A ball of mucus that blocks the entrance to the cervix during pregnancy.

multiples: Expecting two or more babies.

mumps: A viral infection that normally affects the glands beneath the ears and is characterized by severe swelling and pain.

myomectomy: A surgical procedure to remove uterine fibroids.

necrosis: Tissue or cell death.

non-stress test or NST: A test that evaluates the fetus's wellbeing with an electronic fetal monitor by measuring the fetal heart rate.

obesity: A condition where an individual is severely overweight. Characterized by a BMI equal to and greater than 30.

Obstetrics or OB: A branch of medicine and surgery that focuses on pregnancy and childbirth.

obstetrician-gynecologist or OBGYN: A qualified medical practitioner who specializes in pregnancy, childbirth, and the female reproductive system.

oligohydramnios: Abnormally low levels of amniotic fluid in the uterus.

ovary: A structure in the female reproductive system that produces and releases egg cells, and also plays a role in regulating hormones.

ovulation: The process in the menstruation cycle where an egg cell is released.

oxidative stress: A condition that causes less oxygen to be available for cells to use due to increased toxins in the body.

oxytocin: A hormone naturally produced by the brain responsible for bonding with others, contractions during labor and childbirth, and plays a role in milk production.

palpitations: Skipped or fluttery heartbeat.

pelvic area/region: The area of the body that contains the reproductive organs, the urinary tract, and the rectum.

perineum: The stretch between the anus and the vulva.

Pitocin: Synthetic oxytocin.

pituitary gland: A small gland inside the brain that regulates many of the most important hormonal processes.

placenta: An organ that develops during pregnancy to provide the fetus with oxygen and nutrients.

polycythemic: Abnormally high number of red blood cells in the body.

polyhydramnios: Abnormally high levels of amniotic fluid in the uterus.

Postpartum or PP: The time after childbirth.

predisposition: To be more susceptible to.

preeclampsia: See page 171.

prenatal care: Regularly scheduled appointments with the chosen healthcare practitioner during a woman's pregnancy.

preterm: Before week 37 of pregnancy.

progesterone: A reproductive hormone that is chiefly responsible for maintaining pregnancy.

progestin: See progesterone.

prolapse: When an organ or part of an organ changes position and usually protrudes through an opening.

prostaglandins: A type of lipid in the body responsible for inflammation, fever, vasodilation, and blood clotting. They ripen and dilate the cervix in response to contractions.

prostatitis: A condition that causes the prostate to become inflamed.

pruritic urticarial papules and plaques: A rash or itchy hive-like bumps that can form during pregnancy around the abdominal area.

polycystic ovary syndrome: A medical condition that causes cysts to form on the ovaries.

pulmonary embolism: A clot in the lungs.

receptor: A structure inside the body, that when stimulated, causes an effect in the body.

recreational drugs: Chemical substances that are used for non-medical purposes. Most are illegal.

rectovaginal fistula: An abnormal connection between the rectum and the vagina.

Rh factor: An inheritable trait that determines what type of protein is found at the surface of the red blood cells. Can be positive or negative.

RNA: Structures in the body responsible for the coding and decoding of genes, and the expression of genes.

scrotum: A sack of skin that helps the testes to hang outside the body for temperature regulation.

selective estrogen receptor modulator: A class of medication that activates, deactivates, or blocks the estrogen receptors.

selective serotonin reuptake inhibitors: A class of medication that is often prescribed to treat anxiety disorders, depressive disorders, obsessive-compulsive disorders, and other mental health conditions.

septic shock: Shock induced by an infection.

sexually transmitted infections: Infections contracted from having sex with an infected person.

shock: A critical medical condition where the blood pressure drops suddenly, leading to poor blood circulation, can cause organ failure, coma, and seizures. Can lead to death.

sickle cell anemia: A genetic disorder where the red blood cells are abnormally shaped, which causes difficulties in blood flow and oxygen transport.

sperm concentration: The number of sperm.

sperm motility: The ability of a sperm cell to move.

spider veins: A usually harmless condition where red or purplish lines fan out from a central point due to stress on the tiny blood vessels in the body.

spina bifida: A birth defect where the spine does not close properly during early pregnancy.

spinal block: Anesthesia is administered via injection into the arachnoid space of the spine.

spontaneous rupture of membranes: Water breaking.

stillborn: Pregnancy loss after week 20 of pregnancy, or losing a baby during labor or birth.

surfactant: A compound on the surface of alveoli to keep them from collapsing by lowering surface tension.

surrogacy: A process by which a woman agrees to be pregnant with another parent/couple's baby and to deliver that baby.

symptoms: What an individual experiences as the consequence of something else.

systolic: The blood pressure measured when the heart is contracting.

testicle (testes): The male reproductive organ responsible for sperm production and hormone release.

testicular torsion: A condition where one of the testicles rotates and causes the spermatic cord to twist and prevent blood flow to the testicles.

testosterone: A hormone responsible for the male reproductive system and the development of male qualities.

thrombocytopenia: A condition where the number of blood platelets is too low.

ultrasound: A method that uses sound to create images of the inside of the body, usually used during pregnancy to create images of the baby.

umbilical cord: The structure that connects the fetus to the placenta so that nutrients and oxygen may be delivered to the fetus, and waste transported away.

urethra: A tube that transports urine from the bladder to the outside of the body.

urethritis: A condition that causes inflammation of the urethra.

uterus: The womb.

vaginal discharge: Fluids excreted via the vagina, which usually consists of fluid, cells, and bacteria. Can vary in thickness and color (clear to whitish), and normally does not have a strong smell.

vaginal ring: A ring-shaped device inserted into the vagina that provides contraceptive protection.

varicocele: A condition where the veins within the scrotum become enlarged.

varicose veins: A condition where the veins close to the surface of the skin become enlarged, and/or twisted, usually on the legs.

vernix caseosa: A greasy, white layer that coats the fetus around week 19 to protect its skin.

zygote: A fertilized egg cell.